PATIENT

SATISFACTION

Defining, Measuring,

and Improving the

Experience of Care

PATIENT

SATISFACTION

Defining, Measuring, and Improving the Experience of Care

Irwin Press

Health Administration Press
ACHE Management Series

Your board, staff, or clients may also benefit from this book's insight. For more information on quantity discounts, contact the Health Administration Press Marketing Manager at (312) 424-9470.

This publication is intended to provide accurate and authoritative information in regard to the subject matter covered. It is sold, or otherwise provided, with the understanding that the publisher is not engaged in rendering professional services. If professional advice or other expert assistance is required, the services of a competent professional should be sought.

The statements and opinions contained in this book are strictly those of the author(s) and do not represent the official positions of the American College of Healthcare Executives or of the Foundation of the American College of Healthcare Executives.

06   05   04   03   02   5   4   3   2   1

Library of Congress Cataloging-in-Publication Data

Press, Irwin.
    Patient satisfaction: defining, measuring, and improving the experience of care/
    Irwin Press.
        p. cm.
    Includes bibiographical references and index.
    ISBN 1-56793-189-8 (alk. paper)
        1. Patient satisfaction. 2. Physician and patient. 3. Medical care—Quality
        control. I. Title.

    R727.3 .P725 2002
    362.1'068—dc21

                                                                    2002023283

The paper used in this publication meets the minimum requirements of American National Standard for Information Sciences—Permanence of Paper for Printed Library Materials, ANSI Z39.48-1984. ∞ ™

Acquisitions manager: Audrey Kaufman; Project manager: Helen-Joy Bechtle; Text and cover design: Matt Avery

Health Administration Press
A division of the Foundation of the
    American College of Healthcare Executives
1 North Franklin Street, Suite 1700
Chicago, IL 60606-3491
(312) 424-2800

Table of Contents

Foreword

AFTER MORE THAN 40 years as a healthcare professional, I thought I was "tuned in" to the importance of providing quality care to patients and their respective levels of satisfaction. But over the past ten years, I have come to redefine quality care, patient safety, and patient satisfaction in a new and more meaningful way.

The transformation began to occur in the 1980s as the quality movement got underway. Those efforts gave me a whole new perspective as to what constituted quality and the importance of measuring quality in the activities that surround the patient care process. This changed my definition of quality care from one that was narrow and clinically focused to one that was much broader and included clinical outcomes, best practices, patient safety, and, indeed, patient satisfaction.

Like many healthcare organizations, our ability to measure and monitor service activity levels and financial performance was significantly more mature than our ability to measure quality patient care or patient satisfaction. But our understanding of quality and safety measures has been significantly enhanced over the past five or so years. Although we measured patient satisfaction religiously and reported the results every quarter, we clearly lacked the focus that we have today. Our results historically were above average;

however, in the latter part of the 1990s during a period of rapid growth and change, this consistent performance was disturbed. After stepping back and taking a fresh look, we designed and implemented a new service excellence program to honor our value of outstanding service. Within the first year of the new program, patient satisfaction results became outstanding and have remained so over the past several years. These results have allowed us to broaden our focus to important related issues, including the satisfaction of our work force and their retention, and patient safety. The learning curve continues. We are far from producing a finished model, but will continue to evolve a set of quality products and services for our patients and to create a workplace environment that attracts and retains talented associates. Our successes in patient satisfaction have convinced me of the necessity of satisfaction efforts to the creation of a culture of service excellence and the overall success of an organization.

Irwin Press brings his considerable talent and years of experience to *Patient Satisfaction.* The healthcare executives who read this book will not only advance their understanding of the importance of patient satisfaction to healthcare, but also learn new ways to raise the level of service quality to their patients. The book includes extensive action steps that will help readers move forward in enhancing their patient satisfaction efforts. A significant portion of the book is devoted to describing and understanding the process of measuring patient satisfaction and how to use, report, and understand the resulting data. Further, we are reminded that proper methodology is important if we want accurate and reliable results. Extensive instruction in how best to report and compare results and how to extract the potential of the data that is collected is also covered.

The comprehensive nature of the text—defining and understanding patient satisfaction, appropriate and realistic methodology, maximizing use of the data, the role of organizational culture, improvement strategies, and so forth—make it essential, relevant reading for the entire spectrum of those who work in the clinical setting. From frontline caregivers to senior administrators and satisfaction program managers (indeed, any who come in contact with patients); all will benefit from the insights of this groundbreaking book.

In conclusion, this book is a very worthwhile addition to the quality movement in our health care facilities.

Dennis R. Barry
President and CEO
Moses Cone Health System
Chairman-Elect
American Hospital Association

Preface

PATIENT SATISFACTION HAS finally come into its own as a serious part of healthcare. Satisfaction measurement is mandated by the Joint Commission on the Accreditation of Healthcare Organizations. Increasing numbers of state hospital associations, purchasers, and insurers are including patient satisfaction "report card" information in public disclosures of hospital quality. Growing numbers of hospitals are using patient satisfaction scores in decisions regarding staff compensation and bonuses. Nationally and publicly, concern for satisfaction is socially and politically correct.

Of all the reasons for paying attention to patient satisfaction, only one transcends "correctness," accountability, or accreditation standards—quality of care. Patient satisfaction is important because it is a *component* of care as well as an *outcome* of care. When patients are satisfied, both the immediate care and subsequent clinical outcomes are enhanced. At the same time, when the quality of care is high, satisfaction will be measurably high. This "double whammy" should be sufficient to make improving and monitoring patient satisfaction a core concern of every healthcare institution and provider.

But it isn't.

Patient satisfaction still does not occupy its proper place of respect and attention. Many take it for granted as a simplistic concept that only requires common sense to understand and track. When those who believe this make little progress in improving satisfaction, their lack of success is often attributed to the "soft," idiosyncratic, and unpredictable nature of patient satisfaction. Other healthcare professionals who do take patient satisfaction seriously may become frustrated by the lack of clear improvement, and frequently blame the survey.

This book is directed to all who wish to improve the patient's experience and evaluation of care and who are willing to put some sweat equity into the effort. Neither patient satisfaction nor its measurement are simple. If they were, all hospitals would have high patient satisfaction. If merely smiling, introducing yourself, and personally taking patients and guests to their destinations were all that mattered, satisfaction would be universally high. But satisfaction involves far more than these obvious surface tactics.

That's what this book is about—the often-missed factors that underlie patient satisfaction, its measurement, and its management.

The patient is with you for a relatively short time—hours or days. There is no time to educate the patient to understand or appreciate what you are doing; therefore, total responsibility for satisfying the patient lies with *you*. The key to patient satisfaction lies in: (1) understanding the patient; and (2) understanding yourself and your hospital's culture.

This book is also about the issues that underlie the measurement of satisfaction and effective use of the data. Patient satisfaction measurement is not typical "market research." Patients are customers, but they are not like any other customer. All things being equal, they *don't* want to use your services! And when they do, they are easily intimidated by staff and by the complex, strange machinery, techniques, and settings. They are reluctant to bite the hand that heals them. Thus, getting patients to provide objective evaluations of care *and* return a survey requires special methods.

Most chapters end with a list of specific suggestions entitled "Action for Satisfaction." Many chapters include examples of survey results and data analyses that show the usefulness of good satisfaction data. Most hospitals have access to similar data, whether internally or externally generated. These data were drawn from Press, Ganey surveys and reports, but most patient satisfaction survey firms provide similar analyses, and if you do your own programming and data crunching, you can generate similar reports.

Healthcare has changed a lot since 1983, when I first started lecturing on patient satisfaction. The three biggest changes from my perspective are the (1) rise of the concern for quality; (2) empowerment of the patient as consumer; and (3) providers' concern for the bottom line and market share. Patient satisfaction has a major effect on all three. I hope this volume adequately supports your need to deal effectively with these issues.

While a number of specific case studies from specific hospitals about techniques or strategies can be used to improve patient satisfaction, I have tried not to overdo my representation of case studies. The problem with a specific case study is that the issue and action depicted may not be relevant for all readers. Thus, I present these as examples only, to stimulate creative discussion rather than to offer a definitive solution.

This is a very personal book and my biases are likely very apparent. I'm an unflinching advocate for patient satisfaction and a firm believer that it is inextricably linked with the "true" quality of care. The distinction between "technical" and "interpersonal" care, or between "care" and "service" should be laid to rest once and for all. Every one of the patient's experiences in the hospital (those with people, machines, or events) are filtered through the patient's knowledge, personality, prejudices, preconceptions, and culture. These filters determine the patient's ultimate evaluation of the experiences, and this evaluation in turn affects the patient's response to care. Mind and body are not wholly independent entities. What the patient experiences, feels, believes, thinks, fears, and hopes about care cannot be separated from the actual outcome of care. Thus, concern for patient satisfaction must ultimately become a routine part of medical management—a day-to-day concern no less important than infection control and surgical protocols. I suspect that this passion of mine will be very apparent throughout the book!

Acknowledgments

Special thanks to Mel Hall, Dennis Heck, and Carla Peterson for their critical reading of earlier drafts. Thanks to my partner, Rod Ganey, for his wisdom and suggestions. Thanks to Charlene Murphy for her dedication in editing my first drafts. Thanks to Andra for her support and inspiration. Helen-Joy Bechtle and Audrey Kaufman of the Health Administration Press deserve thanks for making the editing process so author friendly. Above all, I am grateful to the Press, Ganey family of hospital clients who continually rejuvenate me with their passion for improving the quality of care.

CHAPTER 1

Why Bother?

So—WHY BOTHER with patient satisfaction? Patient satisfaction can be a core strategy for achieving and sustaining the mission of your institution. Done correctly,

- you will achieve higher quality of care;
- your staff will be more content with their jobs and turnover will be lower;
- you will be more likely to stay financially healthy;
- your competitive position will be strengthened; and
- you will be less likely to be sued.

Patient satisfaction is a hot topic. Everyone pays lip service to it. It's politically correct. The Joint Commission says you have to monitor patient satisfaction, and it can also satisfy ORYX requirements. The NCQA (National Committee for Quality Assurance) requires HMOs to monitor it. Increasingly, purchasing coalitions and businesses will require providers to monitor it. State hospital associations are including it in their public report cards. So you have to do something about patient satisfaction. But what?

In spite of the books, articles, and hype, possibly no element in healthcare is so little understood as patient satisfaction. Many still view it as a soft phenomenon—a "happy camper" index that reflects medically uneducated perceptions as opposed to serious evaluations of "real" quality. Many healthcare professionals still feel that patients may be able to judge "service," but not technical/medical care. If the food's bad, they might rate the whole spectrum of care lower. Service and care are distinct entities, they might contend. Don't confuse the two. Care—direct technical intervention (emphasis on "technical")—is the key. Service is peripheral—interpersonal and experiential. To such professionals, "service" suggests that you're treating customers rather than patients. This insults their professional identity.

Service is often viewed as a matter of personality and amenities. Such views have led to simplistic approaches to dealing with patient satisfaction. Most service-focused programs haven't changed much from the "guest relations" efforts of the '80s (which staff often labeled as "smile school"). Look the patient in the eye when talking. Introduce yourself. Sit next to the patient, rather than stand at the foot of the bed. Be courteous. Be caring (whatever that means). Be prompt. Reduce delays. Keep the soup hot and the carpets clean. Care, on the other hand, is often viewed as having to do with IV hook-ups, medication, treatment explanations, post-op instructions, and other technical/informational interventions.

In truth, the service/care distinction is a red-herring issue. *It's all service and it's all care.* The manner in which care is delivered defines, for the patient, the nature and effectiveness of that care. Timeliness, attitudes, information, explanations, body language, physical touch, contextual sounds and sights—all these factors have an effect on the patient's experience of care.

If patients perceive the carpets to be soiled, or corridor noise excessive, or the nurses less than friendly, will it affect their experience of care? Notice I said "experience" of care, not care itself. Is the difference significant? Can the patient have a bad experience of good care? Or does a negative "service" experience actually diminish the effectiveness of the technical intervention? When the nurse explains (or fails to explain) the IV to a patient who has never had one before, is the explanation an element of service or care? If the nurse is professional yet not particularly friendly or empathetic, does this reflect upon service or care? Could poor explanation or lack of friendliness possibly affect the ease and comfort of the "stick"?

What do patients want from healthcare—technical or service quality? Unless asked directly, they usually won't contribute information about what they want (Baker 1998, 72). In a recent study by the VHA, patients were asked whether "clinical quality" or "service" quality carried more weight in their healthcare decision making. Of the respondents, 32 percent said service was more important; 68 percent ranked clinical quality more highly. When the choices were expanded to include clinical quality, service quality, or *both,* fully 59 percent of the initial 68 percent said they would prefer both, while 32 percent steadfastly continued to stress service over clinical quality (VHA 2000, 19). All things being equal, we all want the highest quality of technical (clinical) care. Technical care is a *necessary* criterion for judging care overall. At the same time, it is only a partial—and thus *insufficient*—criterion for making this judgement.

Patients do judge the quality of clinical care they receive. However, they base their judgements on far more than the technical interventions, many of which they are unaware. Patients cannot judge whether the proper gauge needle is used for the injection, or whether 10 cc is the proper dose, or whether heparin is the proper medication. But patients *can* judge whether the injection hurt more than anticipated, whether the nurse was informative as well as friendly, or whether the doctor listened to the patient's ideas and questions and responded appropriately.

Patients cannot distinguish between the technical merits of full incision versus endoscopic surgery for hernia repair, but they can judge whether the doctor explained the options well. They can judge whether staff were sensitive to their post-op pain or whether friends and visiting family were treated with respect and given satisfactory explanations. Patients are aware of whether sensitive, realistic information was given about care at home after discharge or whether the staff appeared to empathize with the personal hardships that resulted from the physical problem and the hospitalization.

Patients enter an interaction with physicians assuming (at least hoping) they are competent. However, if patients perceive that physicians are not interested in them, or not concerned with good communication or empathy, they doubt the physicians' ability to actually use their full competence (Friedson 1961, 208-209).

Patients would then feel that the care being delivered was not of the highest quality. Moreover, they would likely respond with some level of distrust, resulting in potentially incomplete information exchange and potentially a less than optimal response to treatment. In short, the patient's perception of the physician's technical competence (however based) could actually modify the effectiveness of that competence. Here again service and care are inseparable. The patient's total experience of care defines that care and affects the patient's response to it. That this experience is highly personal actually makes its effect on the patient even stronger (c.f. Goldfield et al. 1999, 430). The interactional and perceptual aspect of the experience and the inclusion of familiar "service" elements as well as technical interventions, makes the experience no less significant as a definer of quality.

Patients' experience and perception of care is expressed and measured as patient satisfaction. Therefore, patient satisfaction is a valid outcome indicator of the quality of the *totality* of care experienced.

THE LINK TO QUALITY

Steiber (1988, 84) reports a solid correlation (.71) between patient satisfaction and overall quality of care. Davies and Ware (1987) find a high correlation between patients' evaluations of the technical quality of their care and clinical experts' judgements of this same care. Nelson et al. (1992) find that patients' and physicians' ratings of hospital quality are highly correlated (.52 to .87). Many researchers also believe that patients are quite capable of judging the technical quality of care (Chang et al. 1984; Gerbert and Hargreaves 1986; Cleary and McNeil 1988).

What is it that allows patients to evaluate technical care? After all, patients are not competent clinicians. The consensus is that patients constantly judge the motives and competence of caregivers through their interaction with them. This judgement is a very personal one, based on perceptions of care being responsive to patients' "individual needs," rather than to any universal code of standards (McGlynn 1997). When these individual needs are perceived as being met, better care results. Lohr (1997, 23) notes: "Inferior care results when health professionals lack full mastery of their clinical areas *or cannot communicate effectively and compassionately*" (emphasis mine). In short, when patients perceive motives, communication, empathy, and clinical judgement positively, they will respond more positively to care. This includes physical and behavioral response to care, not just emotional or "evaluational." Sobel (1995) claims that improved communication and interaction between caregiver and patient improves actual outcome. Donabedian (1988, 1744) notes that "...the interpersonal process is the vehicle by which technical care is implemented and on which its success depends" (see also Corah et al. 1985; O'Shea et al. 1986; Babakus and Mangold 1992). Interpersonal and technical aspects of care are not separate phenomena.

What this boils down to is that patient satisfaction is not only an indicator of the quality of care, but a *component of* quality care, as well. When patients are more satisfied, three things occur regarding trust, stress, and the placebo effect.

Trust Is Enhanced

Enhanced trust results in greater compliance, as well as a greater tolerance of uncomfortable or frightening procedures. The relationship between interaction skills (information giving and taking, empathy, etc.) and compliance are fully documented (c.f. Ware and Davies 1984). Physicians generally are incapable of correctly identifying their compliant and non-compliant patients. Patients do not telegraph compliance (they don't usually voice complaints or question judgements on the spot, either). If patients lack trust in the care, medical management will be more difficult and likely less effective. There can be more complaints about discomfort or fear. Patients will also be more likely to "act out" during procedures. Staff can become frustrated.

Some years ago, I spent a year as visiting professor at a large medical school, attached to the department of psychiatry. I noted that in a majority of instances when medical residents called for a "psych consult," it involved a non-compliant patient who would not follow the doctor's orders. The result was more staff intervention and (in many instances) greater resource utilization and length of stay. Overall, when patients are more satisfied, medical management is easier.

Stress Is Reduced

The relationship between stress and medical complications has been known for years (c.f. Nuckolls et al. 1972; Crandon 1979). On the Press, Ganey inpatient survey we ask patients to rate how well their blood was drawn ("quick," "little pain," etc.). We also ask about the friendliness and courtesy of the phlebotomist. Not surprisingly, the two responses are significantly correlated ($r = .448$; $p < .01$). When the nurse puts a patient at ease, there is less stress, more relaxation of muscles—and an easier stick. Greater satisfaction means lower stress and likelihood of fewer complications.

In a fascinating study some years ago, Sosa (1983) followed a group of women who came to a large indigent hospital to deliver their first babies. All of the women in the study came to the hospital alone, with no husband or other person to accompany them.

They were examined on admission and determined to have had a normal, uncomplicated pregnancy to date. All of the women were provided with standard labor/delivery care, and attended by nurses and physicians performing their normal duties. Half this sample, however, were provided with a "doula" to attend them during their labor and delivery. A doula is a lay attendant who simply sits with the mother, providing friendly interaction and support.

Sosa and his colleagues found that women attended by doulas had significantly shorter labor time and experienced far fewer complications than the women who went through labor and delivery alone. Stress reduction via empathetic interaction was clearly a factor here. With increased stress, medical outcomes may be less satisfactory, and higher costs are incurred because of complications.

The Placebo Effect Is Enhanced

"Placebo" is from the Latin for "I please." Moerman (2000) estimates that on average, 30 percent of any cure is a result of the placebo effect. This effect is emphatically not produced by the procedure itself (the pill or technical intervention). A sugar pill isn't a placebo. The *idea* of the pill and what it can do is the placebo. Every intervention in the clinical setting has the placebo effect, by influencing the patient's perception of care. Information, interaction, perceived motives and attitudes of caregivers, concern for physical comfort, decor, symbols, machinery, medications, treatments— every experience contributes to the intervention. All of these can have an effect on the patient's perception of the quality and effectiveness of care *while that care is being given* (not just after discharge).

Physician enthusiasm, for example, can affect patients' response to treatment. So can a positive attitude. One study of patients presenting with vague symptoms scripted doctors to use two different interactions. Doctors told one group of patients, "I don't know what's the matter with you." Patients in the other group were given a clear but benign diagnosis (e.g. "duodenal inflammation") and told that they needed no further treatment. Two weeks later, 39 percent of the first group reported feeling better. Sixty-four percent of the second group (with a definite diagnosis and prognosis) reported feeling better (Moerman 2000).

Moerman (2000) also cites studies demonstrating that short, frank pre-op discussions by anesthetists about postoperative pain led to significantly less analgesic use and shortened hospital stays for patients undergoing abdominal surgery.

The placebo effect is not limited to interactions with physicians or nurses. *Any* experience the patient has with the institution can exert a placebo effect. This applies to decor and food as well as surgical explanations or the courtesy of the IV nurse. With the placebo phenomenon, the effectiveness of the "active" intervention (the surgery or meds) is automatically enhanced. The two factors are additive, not alternatives. Patient satisfaction is a potent placebo.

In sum, when patients are more satisfied, medical management and outcome are enhanced. Patient satisfaction and "actual" quality of care are not distinct phenomena. When your patients are more satisfied, *they really are getting better care.* Thus, when you measure patient satisfaction, you really are measuring your overall quality of care. Quality of care is defined by its effect on patients, not on its being recognized as such by professional experts.

Patients act on what they think or believe. If they think your institution is high in quality, they'll respond as though it is—regardless of the basis of their judgement.

THE LINK TO EMPLOYEE SATISFACTION

If patient satisfaction were linked only to quality of care, that would be enough to justify its importance. That patient satisfaction is also a factor in staff satisfaction—and vise versa—is an added bonus (Schlesinger and Heskett 1991). Atkins et al. (1996) identified a strong relationship between employee satisfaction and patient intent to return to or recommend the hospital. A preliminary study in 2001 by

Figure 1.1 Relationship of Employee and Patient Satisfaction

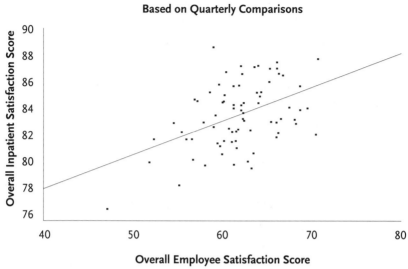

Based on Quarterly Comparisons

n = 76 hospitals that received reports during the same quarter; r = .46; p < .001.

Source: Press, Ganey, Associates. 2001. Preliminary Study.

Press, Ganey of hospitals measuring both patient and employee satisfaction revealed a statistically significant relationship between the two (Figure 1.1).

Quint Studer, CEO of Baptist Hospital in Pensacola, Florida, sees a direct relationship between his employees' satisfaction with their work situation and patient satisfaction with care.

> We tracked both and they rose together. Each affects the other. When patients are more satisfied, staff feel more pride about their jobs and the impact they're having on patients. For their part, patients get better care from staff who like their job and the institution they serve. (Studer 2001)

A key result of staff satisfaction is reduced turnover. Studer reports that from 1996 to 2000, nursing turnover at Baptist dropped from 30 to 13 percent! That, he says, equals $675,000 saved through reduced recruiting and training costs (*Modern Healthcare* 1999, 48).

Similarly, Thunderbird Samaritan Hospital (Glendale, Arizona) reports that nursing staff turnover dropped from 16 to 11 percent from 1998 to 1999 as patient satisfaction made significant gains. Covenant in Lubbock, Texas saw employee turnover drop from 24 to 18 percent (that's actually a 25-percent reduction) over the two-year period in which their satisfaction scores rose significantly.

Like the relationship between satisfaction and quality of care, the patient/staff satisfaction connection is a "natural." The linkage is not quite direct, however. Administrators and policy can act as filters— or catalysts. Where staff are empowered and rewarded for behaviors and strategies that enhance patient satisfaction, staff and patient satisfaction will likely both move upward. If patient satisfaction survey scores become a club with which to threaten staff, and if staff are not rewarded for aggressively addressing identifiable satisfaction issues, both patients and staff may find less to recommend about your institution. If patient satisfaction is high, staff feel more pride in their work and actualize the hospital's mission more enthusiastically. The result is more than mere job approval, of course. When provider satisfaction is high, the result is better medical treatment as well as personal care (Kurata et al. 1992).

THE LINK TO COMPETITIVE STRENGTH

Perhaps because of increasing costs, perhaps because of the growing public familiarity with "customer service" in all other sectors of the economy, patients increasingly view healthcare as a commodity, and they're evaluating it as such. If good service is expected from McDonalds, FedEx, and Nordstroms, it should be expected from the hospital that bills a thousand bucks a day. Good service should also be expected from the health plan for which employees now pay big money. Even well-insured employees are quite aware that they are paying for their own healthcare—either through reduced salaries or bigger deductions from paychecks. Healthcare is a commodity and hospitals and health plans are advertising about as much as local car dealers. Check out the billboards in your town.

Who is the target of the ads, billboards, "fitness walks," women's health festivals, and other publicity-generating programs sponsored by most hospitals these days? The target is individual prospective patients, not physicians. Now, it could be argued that for most employed Americans of all ages, choice of hospital *and* physician are typically limited by the health plans they or their employers select. When my company switched health plans two years ago, the employees were forced to use a different hospital. On the surface, this sounds like the absence of choice. But individual choice and clout are still there.

Good fringe benefits (particularly a decent health insurance plan) are becoming a potent bargaining chip for employers to use in attracting and holding desirable employees. We have very low unemployment in our town. My own company won several key employees away from other local firms because of our health and sick-leave plans. We insure our employees through our health plan, a PPO that offers one of two big local hospitals as the "in-network" provider. If an employee wants to go to the other hospital or other doctors, he or she has to fork over a larger co-payment. How many of my valuable staff have to complain about the company plan's hospital before we decide to dump the PPO for another plan that offers the rival institution? Certainly no more than 10 percent, and probably fewer. When we switched health plans two years ago, it was because the new plan was less costly *and* because eight or ten of our staff of 100 had complained about service at the previous plan's hospital. None of our employees complained about the switch.

When we switched, the previous PPO lost several hundred thousand dollars of business (and they did call us to find out why we took our business elsewhere). The hospital lost far more than that. At the time we switched, it lost 100 insured workers plus their average of 2 to 3 dependents! We now have over 300 insured employees. The lost opportunity cost will total in the millions of dollars over the next four or five years. Cost and employee satisfaction drive our selection of health plans now. We cannot afford a generalized loyalty to any particular hospital. It doesn't matter how many testimonials to their quality that local hospitals publish in the local paper and on local TV or whether a local hospital's name appears among the "best hospitals in the United States" list published by a major national magazine. If enough of our employees don't like the hospital, we will not use it.

Various studies indicate how much financial loss results from a single dissatisfied patient. One patient tells ten or twelve others, these others tell several more, and so on (see TARP 1976; Strasser and Davis 1991, 6-12). By this reckoning, our ten dissatisfied employees turned off more than 120 other potential hospital customers in town. Therefore, the hospital not only stands to lose a lot of money through my company's defection, but additional dollars through negative word of mouth that turns off a substantial number of additional potential customers (Strasser and Davis 1991, 201). The point: Individual patients are gaining unprecedented clout. Dissatisfaction can lead to significant financial consequences for the provider.

If, ultimately, patients are allowed to sue employers for service failures by the company's contracted health plan, many firms will dodge this liability by simply giving up on selecting and offering health plans (and their providers) to employees. Companies will give employees a voucher to purchase their own insurance. These individuals will make their preferences for providers very clear to the health plans that will be competing for their business. Here, patient satisfaction becomes a key to purchase and repurchase. No organization is perfect and hospitals are no exception. However, when customers are highly satisfied, they will be willing to reuse the facility (or another provider bearing the brand identity) even if they have had an isolated bad experience or are bombarded with PR from a competing institution (Oliver 1997, 392). Truly satisfied customers become active "apostles" for the business (Jones and Sasser 1995; Gitomer 1997). Interestingly, studies find that patients are not strongly

Figure 1.2. Percent of Americans Who Say Each Is "Very Believable" in Terms of Providing Information About Quality of Care

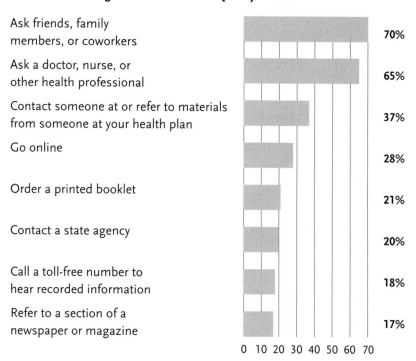

Ask friends, family members, or coworkers — 70%

Ask a doctor, nurse, or other health professional — 65%

Contact someone at or refer to materials from someone at your health plan — 37%

Go online — 28%

Order a printed booklet — 21%

Contact a state agency — 20%

Call a toll-free number to hear recorded information — 18%

Refer to a section of a newspaper or magazine — 17%

0 10 20 30 40 50 60 70

Source: Kaiser Family Foundation/Agency for Healthcare Research and Quality. 2000. *National Survey on Americans as Health Care Consumers: An Update on the Role of Quality Information.* December (conducted July 31-Oct. 13, 2000).

influenced by public claims of quality by hospitals, or by published report cards (Tumlinson et al. 1997; Hibbard and Jewett 1997). Rather, their personal experience and the experiences of significant others has most effect on judgements of quality and decisions to choose one hospital or another (Figures 1.2 and 1.3). Figure 1.2 demonstrates the response when Americans were asked the question, "Who is very believable?" regarding quality of care; Figure 1.3 shows

Figure 1.3 Importance of Familiarity Versus Ratings

Suppose you had to choose between two hospitals

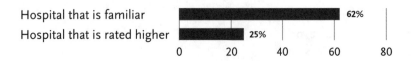

Source: Kaiser Family Foundation/Agency for Healthcare Research and Quality. 2000. *National Survey on Americans as Health Care Consumers: An Update on the Role of Quality Information.* December (conducted July 31-Oct. 13, 2000).

the percentage of Americans who would choose familiarity over ratings.

Ware and Davies (1984, 296) summed it up well: "In addition to delays in care seeking, in the face of serious symptoms, dissatisfaction seems to have other negative effects," including an increase in shopping around for doctors and other providers.

The Brand-Name Phenomenon

The "hospital" is joining the dodo on the extinct list. It is being replaced by the "medical center" and the "integrated healthcare network." To compete for managed care contracts, hospitals have to offer "one-stop shopping," where a single contract will bring the payer a full line of healthcare services. Many hospitals have picked up physician practices, clinics, home health agencies, and diagnostic and surgical centers (to list but a few). All of these are linked through the hospital or medical center name which becomes the "brand" for the entire network. The reputations of all parts of this network are interlinked. Dissatisfaction with any one part can send patients/customers to the competitor (who probably offers a similar range of services). If Mary is dissatisfied with her experience in your emergency department (ED), she might not want to use your outpatient surgical center next year for her hernia repair or your home health agency for her mother. Thus, the financial consequences of dissatisfied customers become multiplied.

A final word about your competition. It's not just the hospital or clinic on the other side of town. Don't forget alternative practitioners. Americans are now spending about as much on chiropractors, naturopaths, massage therapists, nutrition consultants, health food stores, and even the growing supplement sections of their corner pharmacy as they are spending on traditional healthcare. "Technical excellence" does not draw loyalty—and bucks—away from traditional care providers. Most people who use alternative practitioners and practices will tell you that "they treat the whole person" or provide a feeling of greater personal control over one's health. In truth, they provide greater patient satisfaction, not necessarily dramatic medical recoveries.

THE LINK TO PROFITABILITY

The effect of patient satisfaction goes even further. Kenagy et al. (1999) review a number of studies and observe "significant reductions in the costs of care when service improves." In a 51-hospital study, Nelson et al.(1992, 13) found a strong relationship between hospital financial performance and patients' ratings of care. They report that "patient-perceived quality explains up to 30 percent of the variation in hospital profitability. Relatively small increases in the level of patient satisfaction are associated with millions of dollars in year-end earnings for the average hospital" (see also Brown et al. 1993, 13, on potential loss of income to a physician practice that dissatisfies and turns away a single patient). In the largest study of its kind to date, Press, Ganey recently (2002) released findings from 679 hospitals nationwide linking their profitability with patient

Figure 1.4 Patient Satisfaction and Profitability

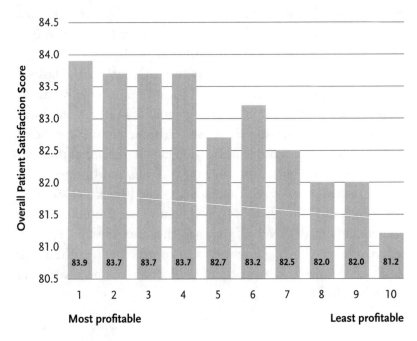

Grouped in deciles based on data from 2001 Medicare Provider Dataset (HCIA) and Press, Ganey 2001 data.

satisfaction. A highly significant correlation was found (r = .23; p < .001) between profit and satisfaction. Data were derived from HCIA's 2001 Medicare Provider Dataset and Press, Ganey 2001 data (Figure 1.4).

Whether patient satisfaction influences financial strength or vice versa remains a question. To investigate this, Press, Ganey (1998) looked at 1997 financial data from over a hundred hospitals reported by HCIA. Patient satisfaction scores from these hospitals were correlated with their profitability and a small statistically significant correlation was found (r = .168, significant at the .05 level). However, the really fascinating and suggestive insight emerged when we looked at these same hospitals' satisfaction scores for the years *prior* to 1997. We found that the 1997 profit figures were more highly correlated with patient satisfaction in 1992 (.269, r = .05) than in 1997! In other words, profitability is more affected by past patient satisfaction than present.

Zimmerman and Skalko (1994, 105) reach the same conclusion: Patient satisfaction is a long-term strategic tool, not just a short-term fix.

This makes good sense. Assuming that the physical problem is dealt with adequately, the patient should have no reason to return anytime soon. Three, four, or five years may elapse before the patient gives the hospital repeat business. In the meantime, he or she is paying continual verbal homage to the institution—which generates additional present-time business.

The question of whether you're treating patients or customers is a red-herring issue. Many healthcare professionals cringe when they hear patients referred to as "customers." They're both. Today's patient is tomorrow's customer. The *patient* experiences care *now*, but selects and patronizes providers *later* as a *customer.*

Of course, a relationship does exist between present satisfaction and present profit. As we suggested earlier, satisfied patients are more likely to respond positively to treatment, with fewer complications, and so forth. This means fewer resources spent and thus a positive financial effect. If hospitals can avoid patient complaints, resources will also be saved. Moran and Malone (1997) conclude that "satisfying patients is more cost effective than responding to complaints."

Interestingly, the link between satisfaction and resource utilization is viewed seriously by some financial institutions. Quint Studer (2001) reports that dramatically improved patient satisfaction scores contributed to Moody's Investor Service's decision to raise Pensacola Baptist's bond rating—a move that cut Baptist's interest payment significantly. Moody's noted that patient satisfaction led to increased market share, which led to increased revenues, which led to a stronger bottom line (Figure 1.5).

Figure 1.5 Moody's Investors Service Rating of Baptist Hospital

Moody's Investors Service

Baptist Hosp., Inc. & The Baptist Manor, Inc. Escambia County Health Facilities Authority, FL.

Moody's Rating   A3

  Issue:
  Series 1998
    Sale Amount $65,000,000
    Expected Sale Date   06/24/98
    Rating Description   Series 1998

Opinion:
A customer satisfaction focus, which permeates the hospital from top management down to floor personnel and whose results now serve as a benchmark for other hospitals, is making a competitive difference and reportedly contributes to some of the 9.8 percent admisssions gain for the year-to-date period ...

Used with permission from Baptist Health Care Corporation, Pensacola, Florida and Moody's Investors Service.

THE LINK TO ACCOUNTABILITY

Everyone's talking about quality, but it's more than talk. An increasing number of external entities want proof of your quality. States are making public lengths of stay, and the number of C-sections physicians perform after vaginal delivery. The National Committee for Quality Assurance's (NCQA) Health Plan Employer Data and Information Set (HEDIS) survey samples a hospital's quality as it taps customers' experiences with their HMOs (after all, the HMO's customers are the hospital's customers). Other agencies, payers, business coalitions, and hospital associations will be issuing "report cards" to the public on your performance (Kenkel 1995). The National Quality Forum is actively attempting to identify an extensive series of outcome measures that will be mandated for all hospitals and the results reported to various public entities. All of these report cards will likely include some form of patient satisfaction measure.

If you look bad on a report card, it can affect your accreditation or your bottom line. An HMO, business coalition, or purchasing group may decide to dump you. At the very least, poor report card scores could force you to renegotiate a contract or settle for reduced payment. Many experts now claim that costs will ultimately begin to level off. The main differentiator between hospitals will be quality or value. I think the key will be value, rather than quality alone.

$$\text{The value equation looks like this: Value} = \frac{\text{Quality}}{\text{Price}}$$

This means that the more you charge, the lower the value you offer your customer. Or, the higher the quality of your care, the higher the value for the purchaser. But what this also means is that higher quality can accommodate higher price and still offer good value. Higher quality can help you strengthen your bottom line.

As a quality measure, patient satisfaction will play a major role. Of course, "hard" clinical indicators such as morbidity, mortality, length of stay, or infection rates are important indicators of quality. They affect the bottom line of health plans and self-insured employers and they must be considered. But patients will increasingly vote with their feet, and their vote is based on their own perceptions of quality. If an HMO, employer, or purchasing group has to choose between two hospitals with relatively similar risk-adjusted clinical outcome figures, patient satisfaction will likely sway the decision. Moreover, lay boards may have little understanding of such indicators as "risk-adjusted length of stay for DRG 237." Everyone understands patient satisfaction, however.

A final note on accountability. Report cards will become more common. Already, state hospital associations are putting pressure on member institutions to measure patient satisfaction (as well as other outcomes) and make these results public. Typically, surveys for report cards are sent out once a year. Moreover, the surveys are relatively short and data are not broken down by nursing unit, shift, department, and so forth. Thus, while the hospital is held publicly accountable for satisfaction scores, the information from these report cards is usually neither timely nor specific enough to allow for identification of problem areas or meaningful targets for quality improvement (QI) efforts. Sporadic public report cards must never be confused with real, ongoing quality improvement instruments. Some hospitals have abandoned regular surveying for QI because they are forced to use report cards, "and we can't afford to maintain two patient satisfaction surveys." Without a QI instrument that is mailed to patients on a consistent basis, no hospital can hope to know its effect on patients and the public—or keep its report card scores up. Discussing the problems of surviving in the report card era, Tu et al. (2001, 10) warn clinicians to "know your outcomes before others do." Ongoing satisfaction monitoring is essential to identifying and addressing internal problems before they show up on external report cards.

THE LINK TO RISK MANAGEMENT

Adding to the competition for patients and contracts, litigiousness among patients is growing. Malpractice insurers (such as St. Paul) are getting out of the business and premiums are on the rise. The unsettling trend in America to view problems, mistakes, and misfortune as "not my fault" is not limited to healthcare. People don't want to accept the consequences of their own behavior. Still less do they want to accept what they perceive as injury from others. Healthcare is different from other purchasable goods or services in that its performance affects one's very life. Americans generally have a sensible attitude toward the limits of performance by most types of professionals for hire, but healthcare is something else. Less than perfect performance can mean disability, discomfort, or death. Healthcare had better be perfect! The medical establishment itself has long fostered this "myth of medical perfection" by refusing to admit the possibility for error or poor judgement ("They might sue us" is the rationale). The growth of malpractice claims is the result.

Patients who are more satisfied are less likely to sue. Period. All studies of malpractice claims show the same result. Communication is the key to the vast majority of suits. Anger, not injury, is the trigger for most claims. Whether the focus is on hospitals or physicians being sued, conclusions are the same: Empathy and good interpersonal skills prevent malpractice claims (Levinson 1994; Levinson et al. 1997; Krowinski and Steiber 1996; Brown et al. 1993, 13; Mock et al. 1995, 14; Troyer and Salman 1986, 384). Typical of these findings is a study of claims among Florida obstetricians (OBS). No relationship was found between prior malpractice claims and present technical quality of the physician. Rather, the authors found that OBS who were sued more often also triggered more complaints of poor interpersonal care. These complaints came from all types of patients, not just those who filed claims (Hickson et al. 1994; Entman et al. 1994).

In truth, suing the caregiver (whether physician or hospital) is something patients prefer not to do. Every risk manager knows that less than 3 percent of reported incidents result in claims. They also know that many claims arise from unreported or imagined incidents. This means that there is a huge emotional component to biting the hand that heals you. Anger or frustration, not shyster lawyers or actual injury, underlie most claims. Even though the average claim never gets to the court stage, it nonetheless costs the provider money via bill write-offs or legal fees.

Elsewhere, I have suggested that dissatisfaction can *negatively predispose* a patient toward the caregivers (Press 1984). A negative predisposition creates a mind-set that encourages the patient to put a more negative spin on both unusual and normal events. When more satisfied, the patient is positively predisposed toward the caregivers and toward events that occur while under the caregiver's control. The following equations make the point:

1. Higher Patient Satisfaction = Positive Predisposition
2. $\dfrac{\text{Positive}}{\text{Predisposition}} + \dfrac{\text{Negative}}{\text{Incident}} = \text{Less Likelihood of Claim}$

What this adds up to is that patient satisfaction is ultimately the most useful strategy for risk prevention. *The cheapest claim to deal with is the one that is prevented because the patient doesn't think of it or want to do it in the first place.*

When Baptist Hospital of Pensacola first thought of instituting a serious patient satisfaction program, their scores placed them as low as the 10th percentile among their national peers. By the end of 1995 Baptist had faced 60 malpractice claims and shelled out more than $200,000 in settlements. A vigorous patient satisfaction program was subsequently implemented. By the end of 1997, Baptist ranked in the 98th percentile nationally. In 1998 only 20 malpractice claims were made, with a total payout of $23,000—an almost a tenfold decrease! Only four claims had been made by the end of the third quarter of 1999. Quint Studer, CEO of Baptist, states that risk management processes themselves had not been altered. The drop in claims was primarily a result of increased patient satisfaction (*Modern Healthcare* 1999, 47). For their efforts, Baptist was MMI/*Modern Healthcare's* 1999 "Excellence in Healthcare Risk Management" award recipient.

CONCLUSIONS

As in many other industries, "product" and "service" are indistinguishable in healthcare. Healthcare, after all, is essentially a service industry, with interaction and intervention (as opposed to a tangible object) constituting the product. The manner in which care is delivered has an effect on outcome—both perceived and physically experienced. From diagnosis to medical management, all aspects of care require sensitive interaction between provider and patient. Decor and amenities, attitudes, professional role behavior, content, and mode of information giving—all these factors have an impact on the effectiveness of and the patient's evaluation of care. Thus, the distinction between "care" and "service" is moot. All care consists of service as well as technical intervention. "Patient satisfaction" is another way of referring to the patient's evaluation of care. Patients continually evaluate and reevaluate care as they experience the hospital, clinic, or physician's office. Because this evaluation has an impact on the effectiveness of care both during and after its delivery, patient satisfaction is a component as well as an outcome and measure of care quality.

Because it is a component of care, patient satisfaction affects medical management and thus, costs. More satisfied patients will use fewer resources and require less time in treatment. As today's patients are tomorrow's customers, satisfaction also translates into market share. And because your patients are also the customers of health plans, higher satisfaction means stronger competitive position (vis a vis managed care contracts). Patient satisfaction also translates into job satisfaction for staff, which in turn can result in lower turnover and more effective recruiting. This is particularly important in an era of chronic nursing shortages. Finally, satisfied patients are less likely to seek legal action as the means to resolve negative issues.

What this all adds up to is that patient satisfaction is an inseparable part of care, quality, and successful healthcare operations. Patient satisfaction is a potent mechanism for increasing and sustaining your quality, efficiency, market share and bottom line. Best of all, efforts to improve patient satisfaction more than pay for themselves. To be a patient satisfaction–driven organization doesn't take big bucks—only commitment.

ACTION FOR SATISFACTION

1. Educate everyone in your organization about the value of patient satisfaction for their mission and for their job security. The overriding characteristic of a patient satisfaction–driven organization is universal commitment by staff at all levels. Commitment comes when staff (especially top management) believe that high patient satisfaction is essential to achieving the organization's mission. Such an orientation does *not* automatically come with the territory; if it did, patient satisfaction would not be an issue today. Education is required. Quite apart from the organizational changes required, staff must be educated in the advantages (for themselves and for their employer) of a patient satisfaction–driven culture. Written material (such as this book) should be distributed to all.

2. Organize discussion groups that focus on the advantages of a patient satisfaction orientation for each specific department or type of staff. Keep the group size modest to encourage interchange. In the discussion groups, each staff member can be required to share with others an example of how their own jobs could be easier, more rewarding, and more secure if patient satisfaction were high. When a number of people share these personal insights (even if some examples appear rather "forced" or tenuously linked to patient satisfaction), it is easier for staff to begin buying into the strategy. If each discussion group consisted of representatives from different departments (including different levels of staff), they might highlight the broad usefulness of patient satisfaction to the overall success of the organization.

REFERENCES

Atkins, P. M., B. Stevenson-Marshall, and R. Javalgi. 1996. "Happy Employees Lead to Loyal Patients." *Journal of Healthcare Marketing* 16: 15-23.

Babakus, E., and W. G. Mangold. 1992. "Adapting the SERVQUAL Scale to Hospital Services: An Empirical Investigation." *Health Services Research* 26: 676-86.

Baker, S. 1998. *Managing Patient Expectations.* San Francisco: Jossey-Bass.

Brown, S. W., A.-M. Nelson, S. J. Bronkesh, and S. D. Wood. 1993. *Patient Satisfaction Pays: Quality Service for Practice Success.* Gaithersburg, MD: Aspen Publishers, Inc.

Chang, B., G. Uman, L. Linn, J. E. Ware, Jr., and R. Kane. 1984. "The Effect of Systematically Varying Components of Nursing Care on Satisfaction in Elderly Ambulatory Women." *Western Journal of Nursing Research* 6 (4): 367-79.

Cleary, P., and B. McNeil. 1988. "Patient Satisfaction as an Indicator of Quality Care." *Inquiry* 25: 25-36.

Corah, N., R. O'Shea, and G. Bissell. 1985. "The Dentist-Patient Relationship: Perceptions by Patients of Dentist Behavior in Relation to Satisfaction and Anxiety." *Journal of American Dental Association* 111: 443-46.

Crandon, A. J. 1979. "Maternal Anxiety and Obstetric Complications." *Journal of Psychosomatic Research* 23: 109-11.

Davies, A., and J. Ware, Jr. 1987. "Involving Consumers in Quality of Care Assessment: Do They Provide Valid Information?" [White paper, December]. Santa Monica, CA: Rand Corporation.

Donabedian, A. 1988. "The Quality of Care: How Can It Be Assessed?" *JAMA* 260: 1743-48.

Entman, S. S., C. A. Glass, G. B. Hickson, P. B. Githens, and K. Whetten-Goldstein. 1994. "The Relationship Between Malpractice Claims History and Subsequent Obstetric Care." *JAMA* 279: 1588-91.

Freidson, E. 1961. *Patients' Views of Medical Practice.* New York: Russel Sage Foundation.

Gerbert, B., and W. Hargreaves. 1986: "Measuring Physician Behavior." *Medical Care* 24: 838-47.

Gitomer, J. 1997. "Your Customer's Happiness Requires Partnering Approach." *Business First* 8: 15.

Goldfield, N., et al. 1999. "The Content of Report Cards: Do Primary Care Physicians and Managed Care Medical Directors Know What Health Plan Members Think Is Important?" *Journal on Quality Improvement* 25: 422-31.

Hickson, G., E. Clayton, S. Entman, P. Githens, K. Whetten-Goldstein, and F. Sloan. 1994. "Obstetricians' Prior Malpractice Experience and Patients' Satisfaction with Care." *JAMA* 272: 1583-87.

Hibbard, J., and J. Jewett. 1997. "Will Quality Report Cards Help Consumers?" *Health Affairs* 16 (3): 218-28.

Jones, T., and W. Sasser, Jr. 1995. "Why Satisfied Customers Defect." *Harvard Business Review* (Nov/Dec): 88-99.

Kaldenberg, D. 1999: "The Relationship Between Patient Satisfaction and Financial Performance." *Satisfaction Monitor* (Nov/Dec): 10.

Kenagy, J., D. Berwick, and M. Shore. 1999. "Service Quality in Health Care." *JAMA* 291: 661-65.

Kenkel, P. J. 1995. *Report Cards: What Every Health Provider Needs to Know About HEDIS and Other Performance Measures.* Gaithersburg. MD: Aspen Publishers, Inc.

Krowinski, W., and S. Steiber. 1996. *Measuring and Managing Patient Satisfaction, Second Edition.* Chicago: American Hospital Publishing, Inc.

Kurata, J., A. Nogawa, D. Phillips, S. Hoffman, and M. Werblun. 1992. "Patient and Provider Satisfaction with Medical Care." *The Journal of Family Practice* 35 (2): 176-79.

Levinson, W. , D. Roter, J. Mullooly, V. Dull, and R. Frankel. 1997. "Physician-Patient Communication: The Relationship With Malpractice Claims Among Primary Care Physicians and Surgeons." *JAMA* 277: 553-59.

Levinson, W. 1994. "Physician-Patient Communication: A Key to Malpractice Prevention." *JAMA* 272: 1619-20.

Lohr, K. N. 1997. "How Do We Measure Quality?" *Health Affairs* 10 (3): 22-25.

McGlynn, E. 1997. "Six Challenges in Measuring the Quality of Care." *Health Affairs* 16 (3): 7-21.

Mock, J., K. File, J. Norwitz, and R. Prince. 1995. "The Effect of Urgency on Patient Satisfaction and Future Emergency Department Choice." *Healthcare Management Review* 20 (2): 7-15.

Modern Healthcare. 1999: "Paying Attention to the Healthcare Consumer." (October 25): 47-48.

Moerman, D. 2000. "Cultural Variation in the Placebo Effect: Ulcers, Anxiety, and Blood Pressure." *Medical Authority Quarterly* 14: 51-72.

Moran, N. Y., and M. P. Malone. 1997. "Utilizing Patient Satisfaction to Meet the Challenges of Managed Health Care." *Home Health Outcomes and Resource Utilization Integrating Today's Critical Priorities,* edited by C. Adams and A. Anthony, pp 1-9. New York: National League for Nursing Press.

Nelson, E., R. Rust, A. Zahorik, R. Rose, P. Batalden, and B. Siemansk. 1992. "Do Patient Perceptions of Quality Relate to Hospital Financial Performance?" *Journal of Health Care Marketing* 12 (4): 6-13.

Nuckolls, K., J. Cassel, and B. Kaplan. 1972. "Psychosocial Assets, Life Crisis and The Prognosis of Pregnancy." *American Journal of Epidemiology* 95: 431-41.

Oliver, R. 1997. *Satisfaction: A Behavioral Perspective on the Consumer.* New York: Irvin/ McGraw Hill.

O'Shea , R., N. Corah, and T. Thines. 1986. "Dental Patients' Advice On How To Reduce Anxiety." *General Dentistry* 34 (Jan/Feb): 44-47.

Press, Ganey Associates. 2002. "Patient Satisfaction and Hospital Profitability: A National Study." [Internal Research Report.] South Bend, IN: Press, Ganey Associates.

Press, Ganey Associates. 1998. "Present Profit and Past Satisfaction." [Unpublished research report.] South Bend, IN: Press, Ganey Associates.

Press, I. 1984. "The Predisposition to File Claims: The Patient's Perspective." *Law, Medicine and Health Care* 12 (2): 53-61.

Schlesinger, L. A., and J. L. Heskett. 1991. "Customer Satisfaction Is Rooted in Employee Satisfaction." *Harvard Business Review* (Nov/Dec): 148-49.

Sobel, D. S. 1995. "Heltialsing Medicine: Improving Health Outcomes with Cost-effective Psychosocial Interventions." *Psychosomatic Medicine* 57: 234-44.

Sosa, R. A. 1983. "Some Observations on Effect of a Supportive Companion During Labor and Delivery." *Journal of Florida Medical Authority* 70: 761-63.

Steiber, S. 1988. "How Consumers Perceive Health Care Quality." *Hospitals* 62 (7): 84.

Strasser, S., and R. M. Davis. 1991. *Measuring Patient Satisfaction for Improved Patient Services.* Chicago: Health Administration Press.

Studer, Q. 2001. [Personal interview] (Feb).

TARP. 1976: "Consumer Complaint Handling in America." [NTIS PB80-196316]. Washington, D.C.: White House Office of Consumer Affairs.

Troyer, G. T., and S. L. Salman. 1986. *Handbook of Health Care Risk Management.* Rockville, MD: Aspen.

Tu, J., I. Schull, J. Ferris, and D. Redelmeier. 2001. "Problems for Clinical Judgement 4: Surviving in the Report Card Era." *Canadian Medical Association Journal* 164: 1709-12.

Tumlinson, A., H. Bottigheimer, P. Mahoney, E. Stone, and A. Hendricks. 1997. "Choosing a Health Plan: What Information Will Consumers Use?" *Health Affairs* 16: 229-38.

VHA. 2000. *Consumer Demand for Clinical Quality: The Giant Awakens.* 2000 Research Series, V.3.

Ware, J., and A. Davies. 1984. "Behavioral Consequences of Consumer Dissatisfaction with Medical Care." *Evaluation and Program Planning* 6: 291-97.

Zimmerman, D., and J. Skalko. 1994. *Re-Engineering Health Care.* Franklin, TN: Eagle Press.

CHAPTER 2

The Basics

PATIENT SATISFACTION IS a summation of all the patient's experiences in the hospital. Satisfaction can be rated high or low. When we talk of increasing or improving patient satisfaction, we are talking about enhancing the experience of care, resulting in a more positive patient evaluation.

WHAT IS BEING EVALUATED?

As suggested earlier, for patients, "service" translates into "care," and service consists of many different types of interactions and experiences.

Customer service circles speak of "moments of truth." In healthcare, these moments essentially refer to any experiences that can have an effect on the patient's predisposition toward the caregiver. The experiences can be mundane, positive, or terrifying: A dirty floor; a surprisingly tasty dessert; a receptionist who talks on the phone, oblivious to the patient standing next to the desk; a physician leaving the room before the patient fully understands the explanation or instructions; empathy and clear explanations from the nurse as she inserts a catheter; an unkept promise that the doctor would be back in 10 minutes.

Imagine the hundreds of sights, sounds, impressions, events, and interactions that every patient experiences in your hospital—from the first glimpse of your sign and the entrance to the parking lot to the functioning of the lobby door at the moment of discharge. Actually, the patient's experience often begins even earlier, with the physician practice (that you may own or contract with), or in the outpatient clinic, lab, or radiology department of the hospital where pre-admission testing is done.

All interactions and experiences in the hospital are potential moments of truth. The patient does not recognize a meaningful distinction between technical and interpersonal experiences. To complicate matters, the number of experiences that form an evaluation could almost be doubled because experiences of family and friends affect the patient's overall evaluation of the institution and the care. Patient satisfaction is most often a result of consensus, rather than a solitary evaluation by the patient alone. Spouses and children can have significant input into the patient's evaluation of care. Indeed, in many instances the spouse or mature child fills out the patient satisfaction survey. As the baby boomers age, this second-hand evaluating is going to happen more frequently.

An experience becomes a moment of truth if it is particularly positive or negative and thereby makes an impression. The incoming patient and her husband ask a housekeeping employee directions to the nursing unit, and are escorted in person. The patient and spouse are positively affected. The OB resident in Labor and Delivery repeatedly passes the bed of the young single mother-to-be, and never stops to give a few friendly words of encouragement or to reassuringly squeeze her foot. The mother doesn't consciously expect a foot squeeze, so she doesn't really note its absence, but an opportunity for a positive "moment of truth" has been missed. Again, any act of omission or commission can affect patient perceptions. Singly in some cases, collectively in others, these acts can have a significant impact on the patient's overall evaluation of, and (as we noted earlier) response to, care.

Since any experience could have a conscious effect on the patient, producing a definitive list of all potential "moments of truth" is impossible—let alone coming up with suggestions for making a positive experience of each moment. Moreover, all hospital experiences are not equal. A dirty floor, poor signage, or cold soup can affect patient satisfaction with the overall hospital experience, but these are not the same as a painful IV start or poor information about a scary-sounding test. Nor do these details have the same effect on patients as does staff inattention to the social and emotional experience of sickness and being hospitalized.

In general, the following rank ordering holds for the inpatient experience.

(a) Good food counts more than lousy food.
(b) Friendliness counts more than good food.
(c) Communication counts more than friendliness.
(d) Empathy enhances communication.

Analogous elements hold for emergency, outpatient, and all other patient contacts within the clinical setting. The comfort and cleanliness of the emergency waiting room are more significant than food. Friendliness is always important. Communication is always important, and empathy makes communication more effective. In the ED, waiting time becomes an important issue, but as we shall discuss later, good communication (explanations for delays) can significantly mitigate the effect of waiting time.

Notice that technical quality is not mentioned in the hierarchy above. That is because it is *assumed*. IV drip rates, appropriateness of medications, appropriateness of surgical technique used—all are issues of technical quality that patients typically do not perceive or evaluate. Ask anyone what she wants of a visit to the doctor or hospital and you will get a pretty consistent answer: "Competent diagnosis and/or cure." If asked whether they would forgo this for friendliness, communication and empathy, most would give a resounding "No!" This being said, we must emphasize once again that patients do judge your technical quality, but base their perceptions on interactions and experiences that could be described as "service" issues. These issues are encompassed in the list above.

Of course, this hierarchical listing is simplistic. Communication is important, but what should be communicated? *What* should staff empathize with? Even "good food" is not a simple issue. Does a Cambodian or Japanese migrant feel comfortable eating a first-quality though "standard" American breakfast of eggs, hot cakes, sausages, and coffee? Good food is not necessarily "appropriate" food. Will a rural Mexican migrant with severe dehydration and diarrhea (a "cold" disease) feel confident about the sensitivity and quality of care if orange juice (a "cold" food) is offered with a meal? "Everyone" knows that cold foods can make cold diseases worse! Only opposites can cure.[1]

All of this suggests that patient satisfaction is far more complex than is commonly assumed.

EXPECTATIONS AND HOPES

We must be realistic. Patients do not have expectations about all aspects of clinical care. Some patients have past experience with the acute care setting, others have none. Even those with prior clinical experience may not be in the hospital for the same procedures and interactions with the same types of staff. Thus, no patient comes to the clinical encounter with a complete set of clear expectations about care. First-timers may bring few specific expectations to the hospital. They may expect that registration will be efficient and easy, but they will probably have no preconceived idea about what occurs during registration or why certain questions are asked. Patients may "know" about ivs, but beyond hoping that it will be relatively painless, may have little idea of who usually does it, precisely where the needle is inserted, or what the drip rate indicates.

I remember the first time I had an IV. First, I was appalled and sickened by the needle being inserted into the back of my hand. That's not a natural place to stick a needle! What if I moved my hand, and the needle wiggled about? It would pierce the vein and I'd bleed to death! Later, the fluid in the clear plastic bag was running out. I had seen enough B movies and TV whodunnits to know that you can kill someone by injecting air into a vein. I pounded the call button vigorously. The nurse took forever to answer the call (almost 5 minutes—an eternity when death was so imminent!). She informed me that the machine next to the bed (the drip-regulating mechanism) prevents any air from getting into the vein, and that the IV would be automatically shut down if the fluid ran out. The information calmed me, but not before I'd spent those terrifying minutes with my ignorance. I also felt somewhat embarrassed. After all, I was a college professor and should have known about the IV. I felt that I'd made a fool of myself. I also felt that I'd been taken for granted. That's not very satisfying. Afterwards, if I'd gotten a patient survey in the mail, I'd have rated the technical quality of the IV as no more than a 3 on a 5 point scale. I've subsequently had several other IVs and can say that in retrospect that first stick was probably closer to 5 in technical competence. But this is immaterial, because I had already complained to family and friends about that first IV.

I'd come to the hospital with no IV experience (or clear expectations about IVs), yet felt quite capable of evaluating it both during and afterward. Having no prior experience with clinical care doesn't mean the patient lacks a basis for evaluating it. Each event stimulates an evaluation by the patient.

Expectations are assumptions of performance. They are based on:

1. Past clinical experiences of self and significant others.
2. Logic ("It should be done this way"). Note: "Logic" is

also informed by family, community, and cultural values.

3. Custom ("It's usually done this way").

In other words, expectations are essentially evidence based. A patient's expectation about care suggests an element of control ("at least you know what to expect"), even where the expectation is negative ("the cortisone shot will probably hurt"). Because expectations anticipate a certain level of performance quality, merely meeting a positive expectation will not ordinarily result in highest patient satisfaction. If you expect empathetic, skilled, knowledgeable, informative nursing—and get it—you will be satisfied, but not necessarily "wowed." You'll think, "It's what should have happened in the first place." When expectations of any kind are met (no matter how positive) the result is no surprise; the care is "appropriate," but not "special."

Expectations, of course, can be positive or negative. If you expect the hospital food to be lousy—and it is—you won't be satisfied. This is why asking survey questions about whether expectations were met does not work. Assume on a survey you are asked how well nursing met your expectations and how well the food service met your expectations. Assume you expected great nursing and lousy food. Assume you got both. You'd give both issues high marks for meeting your expectations!

Any expectation—even a negative one—is useful in that by simply thinking you know what to expect (even if it is pain), uncertainty is minimized and stress can be anticipated and controlled. However, meeting negative expectations does not mean you are satisfying your patients. Things may be more predictable, but certainly not more pleasant.

Meeting or surpassing different kinds of expectations can have different implications:

- Positive performance expectations met = satisfaction
- Positive expectations surpassed = higher satisfaction

- Negative expectations met = dissatisfaction
- Negative expectations surpassed = satisfaction to highest satisfaction

When negative expectations are surpassed, patients are being positively surprised or delighted. Negative expectations are always accompanied by *hopes*. Hopes are wishes, not anticipations of performance. You don't expect them to be met. Hopes differ significantly from expectations in that hopes are based on a lack of knowledge and reflect fear and uncertainty.

For example, you are led to a treatment cubicle in the ED; you *expect* a delay (you've heard lots of horror stories about EDs), but you *hope* the doctor will come in quickly. In another instance, you come in for your first cortisone shot in your elbow; you *expect* it will hurt; you *hope* it won't. You expect mediocre hospital food; you hope it will be acceptable (you don't even hope for delicious!). On the other hand, you expect competent, empathetic nurses. No hopeful thinking is involved here, the nurses had better be good.

For many of the experiences and events they will encounter, patients (particularly first-timers) have no clear expectations—only hopes that

- Staff will be competent.
- Treatment will be fast.
- Treatment will not be uncomfortable.
- Treatment will be effective.
- The patient will be out quickly.
- The patient will feel better.

Hopes tend to be more idealized and simplistic than expectations, and are quite often unachievable. However, because hopes are idealized, satisfaction is automatically high when hopes are realized.

Thus, clinical staff must have some idea about patients' expectations and hopes regarding their clinical experience. Expectations are more specific than hopes. To at least some extent, they are based on past healthcare experience (of the patient or others) and logic (rational business practices, consumer orientation). Ostensibly, therefore, hospitals should find it easier to meet expectations than hopes. When you know patients' expectations you are in a better position to modify your technical, informational, or organizational performance. Expectations may also require special explanations to foster a more realistic understanding of the limitations of clinical care.

Hopes, on the other hand, being idealized and general, require reassurance, support and empathy, as well as explanations about anticipated aspects of care. Providing what the patient hopes for may be impossible. Recovery from knee surgery is never painless, despite a patient's hopes. So long as the patient knows that your intentions are to realize what they hope for, but that the realization of the hope may be thwarted by the limitations of medicine or hospital organization (not your personal limitations—that only creates dissatisfaction with the quality of the staff!), patients will be forgiving and understanding. And satisfied with the care they do receive.

Staff should elicit patient expectations and hopes prior to any procedures, prognoses, or discussions of disease management. By knowing what patients expect or hope, you can deal with erroneous conceptions or clarify your limitations before a perfectly "normal" but unsatisfactory experience occurs.

SATISFACTION AS A PRODUCT OF INTERACTION BETWEEN TWO CULTURES

Patient satisfaction is a product of what *both* participants (the patient and the caregiver) bring to the clinical encounter. Patient satisfaction is not a one-sided product of the hospital and its staff, of proper clinical procedures, and basic courtesy. Patient perceptions of care are always filtered through a cloak of culture, experiences, hopes, and expectations. Thus, although communication and empathy are important, *what* to communicate and *what* to empathize with is not necessarily obvious or common sense. Patients, not clinical staff, define the content and performance criteria for satisfying care. Staff must understand something about the patient if satisfaction is to progress beyond a basic level of experience with simple service factors such as food, housekeeping, decor, and common courtesy.

Patients' primary needs are broad based and certainly not merely "service" focused. These needs include accurate diagnosis; information about the condition, procedures, and prognosis; comfort during and after the procedure (be it medical or surgical); clear, realistic discharge instructions and—last but most important—cure; if no cure, at least some hope. Patients want to be taken seriously both as patients and as real people whose family and social and economic lives have been threatened or disrupted by the medical problem and by the isolation and disorientation of hospitalization. Smiles, eye contact, courtesy, and ethnically sensitive food may help, but they are not the primary reason for the patients's presence in your stress-inducing institution. Remember, all things being equal, patients would rather *not* use your services! More preferable places exist for nice decor, smiling folks, and good chow.

To achieve sustained, exceptional patient satisfaction, go beyond the generic service issues. Understand that the interaction between our medical system and the patient is an interaction of cultures, each of which is incompletely known to the other.

Certainly, patients in an industrialized society are part of the wider culture. They are committed to modern medicine—both official and popular. In medical anthropology, we refer to our modern medical system as a "closed" system. This means that in our system, body and self are largely unrelated; health is independent of the patient's moral, social, religious, and economic life. That is, sickness is not a punishment, but a naturally occurring mechanical event. Lifestyle may affect susceptibility, but does not directly cause most diseases. You don't get VD because you've sinned, but rather, because you contracted a virus. Gall stones, prostate cancer, heart attack, or phlebitis are impersonal diseases, largely unrelated to the patient's identity, reputation, and behavior toward others. One's religious, economic, family, social, or political behavior is not a sufficient cause of disease. Our medical system is amoral, impersonal, and mechanical. Cure is also impersonal, mechanical, and universal. "Universal" refers to the fact that a particular disease (syphilis, for example) has the same cause and cure for all patients, regardless of who they are.

The average patient's medical system, on the other hand, is "open." To most of us, sickness is never an impersonal, anonymous event. Body and self are closely allied. Disease threatens one's identity and economic and social obligations (and perhaps one's very existence), and its effect is *always* personal and always has implications for all other aspects of the individual's life. Every instance of sickness calls our strength, competence, and attractiveness into question. These beliefs and feelings can have a significant effect on the patient's expectations of and response to care.

In addition to anxieties and threats to roles and identities, patients bring a complex baggage of beliefs (about health and sickness), expectations (about healing and healers), and misconceptions (about hospitals and treatment) to the clinical encounter. The encounter is further complicated by its occurring in a strange, unintelligible, uncontrollable context—the hospital, physician's office, or clinic.

All of this constitutes "patient culture" and it is brought by every patient to the hospital or physician's office.

It would be easy at this point to summarize by saying that clinicians must know something about patient culture to maximize satisfaction and the quality of care, but it's not that simple. If patients' personal beliefs, anxieties, and expectations can influence their experience and evaluation of care, so too can clinical culture influence that experience. An understanding of "where the patient's coming from" is insufficient if this knowledge is filtered through a clinical culture that itself impedes accommodation of the patients' needs. If patients' beliefs, expectations, anxieties, and personal issues are "understood" yet viewed by staff as illegitimate, erroneous, or irrelevant, the result will be missed opportunities for reassurance and optimization of care. To satisfy patients, you must know something about yourself as well as them.

Thus, it is imperative that staff recognize their own culture. Clinicians bring an equally complex baggage of beliefs, expectations, misconceptions, family roles, prejudices, professional and personal identities, organizational culture, and hospital roles to the encounter with patients. Staff professional values, for example, can lead to lack of respect for patients presenting complaints. Harried emergency department staff may roll their eyes when a parent with a "snivelly nosed kid" demands immediate attention. Here, a professional trained to deal with major trauma could feel abused by patients who present with "inappropriate" complaints. Such values (prejudices, or whatever you might call them) might be expressed behaviorally through do-the-minimum examination and interaction that are adequate, but no more than that. This attitude can be sensed by the patient.

Organizational rules can also affect staff sensitivity to patient needs. For example, documentation is essential for many reasons: continuity of care from shift to shift, coordination among different staff and specialties, to meet external regulatory requirements, to establish a "paper trail" for risk management, and so forth. Regardless of their functionality, paperwork requirements can result in slower staff response to patients. No matter how firmly we argue that paperwork is a necessary part of care, patients don't see it this way. Paperwork is not the hands-on care that patients want or that they base their evaluations on but appears to be an optional, ostensibly postponable activity that takes staff time away from direct patient care. In other words, paperwork is a part of hospital culture (and thus amenable to modification), not part of the technical act of healing.

CONCLUSIONS

All things being equal, patients never, ever want to use your services.[2] When they do enter your hospital they are not there for the food, decor, or company. They are there for the serious business of diagnosis and/or cure. Patients' familiar routines, timetables, and social and economic identities (if not their very lives) are threatened by the sickness and hospitalization. Under these circumstances, any event or interaction (including the surroundings, machinery, etc.) experienced while under the hospital's care may significantly influence the patient's response to and evaluation of that care.

Of course, familiar service issues (friendliness, timeliness, surroundings) are important because they are among the most familiar and intelligible issues the patient experiences in the hospital. These services are necessary but insufficient for high patient satisfaction. Patient and hospital represent two very different cultures. To achieve high levels of patient satisfaction, hospitals must progress beyond these "low-hanging fruit," to learn more about both patients and themselves. Each represents a culture with its own values, expectations and behaviors. Clinical staff must learn more about the effect of sickness and hospitalization upon patients' personal lives and their experience of healthcare. At the same time, staff must learn more about their own culture—the personal and professional rules, values, and habits that affect their evaluation of and response to patients.

ACTION FOR SATISFACTION

1. Assume the following:
   a. The patient is a stranger in a strange place.
   b. Patients know nothing about the hospital and its rituals and routines.
   c. Patients will easily misinterpret what you are doing or saying.

d. Patients are constantly judging your hospital and the performance of every individual with whom they come in contact.

e. Every experience has some effect on the patient's evaluation of care.

2. Work with staff at all levels to develop an orientation toward patient satisfaction. So many things happen to the patient that it is impossible to specify appropriate tactics for dealing with individuals in specific situations. Familiarize staff with the five assumptions above and initiate discussion about how best to respond to each.

3. Encourage staff (from the CEO down) to develop an orientation that views the hospital as their home and the patients as guests. Would you be continually friendly toward house guests in spite of your own worries or stresses? Would a guest be left wandering in a hallway without someone asking if help or information is needed? Would you pass by a gum wrapper on the floor of your home without picking it up? Would you serve a meal and not ask if there were something else the guest might want? Would you barge into the guest's room without knocking? The guest/home orientation is a general one that, if actively exhibited (and rewarded by administration!), will cover a myriad of situations—including unpredictable ones.

4. Second-guess your patients. Assume that they know nothing about what is being done, yet want to. Staff must be encouraged to imagine questions that patients might have about procedures and events, and discuss explanations that could answer these questions— ideally before questions are asked. Assume that patients have expectations about care that differ from yours and that your motives and actions will be misinterpreted. With the guest/home model and with the significance of information and explanation in mind, the opportunity exists to create and exceed expectations during the patient's stay.

5. Elicit patients' expectations and hopes about their treatment. Devise strategies to meet the expectations or explain why they cannot be met.

6. Examine your own culture for roadblocks to sensitive care. Have staff identify rules and regulations that could affect patients receiving timely, efficient, sensitive care. Start by asking staff to identify "really stupid" rules.[3] This is fun and focuses analytical attention on the often arbitrary nature of regulations. Then, expand the focus to rules that are "logical," yet that may be nonetheless arbitrary. For example, some hospitals require that only nurses be permitted to pass meal trays. The rationale is that only nurses know what patients should or should not be eating, and that if food service staff were allowed to pass trays, serious health-endangering errors could result.

Given that many hospitals allow food service staff to pass trays (without endangering patients), a good discussion could result in reevaluation of rules that impede timely service. A similar rationale lies behind a common rule that only nurses be allowed to respond to patient call buttons. Some hospitals require that the staff member closest to the patient's room (regardless of that person's job in the hospital) respond to the call. A nurse is notified if required. Often the patient wants some service that anyone could provide and this saves time for busy nurses. Discussions about such rules can lead to increased sensitivity toward hospital practices that often result from turf protection rather than sound patient care needs.

7. Organize workshops in which staff examine their attitudes toward patients. Attempt to identify categories of "problem" patients (by payer, by ethnicity and race, by type of medical problem or procedure, by personality characteristics, and so forth). Are these feelings based on stereotypes or consistent experiences with these types of patients? Discuss why such attitudes exist and what their potential effect could be on style of interaction with patients and on medical management decisions. How can such attitudes be modified

while at the same time recognizing that some types of patients do indeed cause emotional or organizational problems for staff?

NOTES

1. In many rural areas of Mexico, ancient humoral medicine beliefs are still strong. Foods, diseases, and medicines are defined as either "hot" or "cold"—categories having nothing to do with actual temperature. Opposites cure, so if one suffers from a cold disease, a hot medicinal is required. Penicillin, for example, is "cold." An anthropologist colleague of mine tells of Mexican patients in a Texas hospital who refused to take penicillin for diarrhea, but found it acceptable if mixed with chocolate (a "hot" substance"), which combated the coldness of the penicillin.

2. An exception may be childbirth. After the birth (and particularly if the new mother stays for several days), the woman is far more a customer than a patient. For some women, the day or two in the hospital is a time for being pampered and a time to gather courage before plunging into the responsibilities of child care at home without skilled nurses and physicians hanging about.

Childbirth is ostensibly a happy, celebratory occasion. The more memorable a hospital can make the experience, the more likely the mother is to think of returning when and if some future medical need arises. The maternity unit offers a prime marketing opportunity for the hospital.

3. The Disney Institute uses the terms "red" rules and "blue" rules. Red rules can never be broken, and there are not many—no smoking around oxygen, for example. Blue rules are hospital operational rules and can be changed.

CHAPTER 3

Digging Deeper:
Patient Vs. Clinical Cultures

PATIENT SATISFACTION DERIVES from the patient's evaluation of how well the provider meets his or her personal and emotional as well as physical needs.

Sending your staff to "smile school" will have only a modest effect on your patients' satisfaction. Patients bring a complex cultural baggage to the clinical encounter. Our closed medical system, as defined in the last chapter, does not typically recognize other parts of the culture as direct causes or symptoms of sickness. Indeed, clinicians can easily recognize such cultural manifestations as "noise."

Patients, on the other hand, work with an eclectic, "open" system of medicine. Although U.S. patients typically "believe in" modern medicine and its impersonal, mechanical paradigm of causality and cure, the effect of disease on a patient is *anything* but impersonal and mechanical. Roles and identities are threatened. Moreover, as disease disrupts lives and lifestyles—or at the very least our daily plans—patients have coping mechanisms for dealing with symptoms, sickness, and disability. In other words, all patients come to the hospital with their own medical system. Those who work in the clinical setting should have some idea of the complexity of this system, because true patient satisfaction derives from the interaction of patient culture and clinical culture.

At first, the discussion that follows might seem more appropriate for physicians than for others in the clinical setting. Not so. Patients' medical beliefs, habits, and personal histories can affect all interactions with all staff. Given that physicians have less contact with patients than dietary or housekeeping personnel (let alone with nurses, technologists, and therapists), the job of understanding "where the patient's coming from" belongs to everyone.

ILLNESS VS. DISEASE

Medical anthropologists (who study the cultural components of sickness and healing) find it extremely helpful to conceptualize the difference between medical and patient cultures as a difference between *illness* and *disease* (c.f. Kleinman et al. 1978).

Disease can be defined as biomedicine's definition of sickness and the physical impact and manifestation of sickness.

Illness can be defined as the patient's definition and view of sickness and the social and emotional effect and manifestations of sickness.

Here, "sickness" is the neutral term. Because patients always have some ideas about their physical problem, and because there are always emotional and social costs to being sick, every case of disease is typically accompanied by an illness. Disease and illness may vary independently. As the patient is treated, effects of the disease may dwindle. At the same time, anxiety about the disease, about missed work, unkept obligations, future health, and so forth, may increase. These concerns form part of the illness. The illness includes all of the effects of the sickness, not just those that are physically sensed. Illness may thus exist in the absence of disease. Illness is always personal. Its effects happen to you and threaten your self-image and identity—whether that be as a superwoman, provider, spouse, professional, or dependable friend.

A large part of patient satisfaction results from the hospital and its staff addressing the patient's illness as well as the disease. A dramatic gap can exist between the two. "To state it flatly," says Eisenberg, "patients suffer 'illnesses'; physicians diagnose and treat 'diseases'" (1977, 11). By recognizing and responding to the illness, providers can go beyond the usual service issues to significantly enhance the patient's experience of care.

EVOLUTION OF AN ILLNESS

An in-depth analysis of the evolution of an "illness" might help to clarify the concept. The interaction with the physician or the treatment in the hospital is merely the last phase of a highly complex process.

Symptoms

Illness begins with the sensation of symptoms. What is a symptom? Not every sensation of pain or discomfort is necessarily defined as a "symptom." I ask students in my clinical anthropology class if any of them has experienced pain or discomfort in the previous several days. Over half raise their hands. One says she had a bad headache that morning. Why didn't she go to the student health service? "Because I was out partying last night and it's just a hangover." Another says he has pain in his left lower back. Why not see a doctor? "Because I was playing basketball yesterday and I'm just stiff. It'll be OK." Perhaps the kid really is merely "stiff," as he suggests, or perhaps he has a major kidney problem. Perhaps the young lady has got a tumor. The point is, neither of them interpreted the discomfort as a "symptom" worth worrying about or bringing to the attention of a professional.

We constantly sift "symptoms," ignoring or downplaying some, paying attention to others. Each of us has a pain or other odd sensation daily. We ignore it, or pop an aspirin and forget it. Studies have indicated that blue collar workers tend to ignore joint and muscle pains. They're "just part of the job."

Pain has a large cultural component. Most humans, regardless of race or ethnicity, have pretty similar pain sensitivities. Notice I did not say "pain thresholds" or "tolerances." That's where culture comes in. Studies indicate that people can take more pain when in the company of their significant others. Pain experienced and tolerated during a tough basketball game with one's buddies might cause a disabling (and illness-identifying) response if the same level of pain occurs when one is alone. Suggestion, too, can affect pain tolerance. In a fascinating study of pain, Lambert et al. (1960) selected a panel of Protestant and Jewish students at a large university. Individually (in private) he tested the pain tolerance of each student and found few differences. After establishing baseline tolerances for each student, he then told half the Protestant subjects (again, individually in private) that Jewish kids can take more pain than Protestants. The other half he told that Jewish kids can take less pain. He did the same with the Jewish students, telling half that Protestants can take more pain and half that Protestants can take less than Jews. Then he retested all the students, again in private. Both groups of Protestant students increased their pain tolerance. The Jewish group that were told they could take less pain than Protestants also increased their pain tolerance. But the Jews told they could take more pain than Protestants stayed relatively stable in pain tolerance. Apparently they didn't want to appear "different."

Pain *tolerance* is but one culturally mediated aspect of pain. *Expression* of pain is another. Zborowski's (1952) classic study of Italian, Jewish, and "old American" patients is a great example. In his study he found that Italian and Jewish patients complained more to nurses about pain. The old Americans (defined as third-generation Anglo-Protestants) complained far less. He concluded that to Italians and Jews, sickness was the cue for a social drama. Complaining about pain was expected in their cultures, and rewarded by nurturant behavior. For the old Americans, sickness was something private and reflective of personal weakness. By minimizing complaints, they felt they were calling less attention to their lessened state.

I came across a clear example of culturally mediated pain expression during my year as a visiting professor at the University of Miami School of Medicine. The obstetric ward at Jackson Memorial Hospital is an ethnic boiling pot. Women of each group express pain differently during labor. I noted that Cuban women tend to complain more when their husbands are within hearing distance. The noise diminishes significantly when only their mothers are present. I remember one young Anglo resident getting quite upset at a Cuban woman in labor, who made a lot of noise while her husband lingered visibly at the doorway. The resident yelled at her, telling her not to "be such a baby." When the husband left, the woman quieted down.

Here, the Cuban woman's expressions of pain serve an important purpose. In a male-dominated culture, childbirth is one of the few areas controlled by the female. By expressing pain, the woman appears to be both victim and hero to her husband. The medical resident's insensitivity to this (as well as the nurses' and doctors' resentment of the complaining Jewish and Italian patients in the previous example) tells patients that the staff "don't really care." The staff, for their part, tend to have their own expectations of what constitutes an "appropriate" amount of pain expression for any given condition. Too much complaint can be disruptive, it becomes noise and can be resented. Patients can sense this resentment. They can be made to feel that they're doing something wrong. This is dissatisfying.

Validating Symptoms

For some patients, being sick means that certain symptoms should be present. For example, French patients typically believe the liver to be a major locus of health and disease. Being sick means having something wrong with the liver. Thus, a French patient who is ill will likely complain of "liver" in addition to any other symptoms that may be felt. When I was working with patients in Bogota, Colombia, almost every hospitalized patient complained about "pain in the mouth of the stomach" in addition to any other symptoms. Such pains constitute a common "validating symptom" in Colombian culture. If you complain of "pain in the mouth of the stomach," it validates for others that you're really sick.

In a fascinating study of such validating symptoms, Zola (1966) focused on Italian and Irish patients at an eye clinic. Although they came largely for *eye* problems, Irish patients tended to complain of discomfort in nose and throat areas as well. Italians, on the other hand, even when they had an eye or ear disorder, "did not locate their chief complaints there, nor did they focus their future concern on these locations." Here, again, each ethnic group expresses illness through special reference to culturally determined parts of the body—not necessarily those parts that reflect the presenting complaint.

I observed a great example while doing research in a large U.S. urban outpatient clinic.

A little old Jewish lady came in to the young resident's office.

Doctor: "How are you doing, Mrs. Goldstein? What's the problem?"

Patient: "Doctor, I'm veak 'n dizzy, I have a svelling in the leg and a pain in the enkle."

Doctor: "How long have you had this swelling, Mrs. Goldstein?"

He asked her a few more questions about the leg, examined her, and determined that she was probably suffering from phlebitis. He wrote a prescription and sent her off.

Afterwards, I asked him if he recalled exactly what Mrs. Goldstein had said as she presented her symptoms. "Sure," he replied. "She said she had a pain and 'svelling' in the leg."

"No,' I corrected. "She started out by saying she was 'veak and dizzy.'"

"Oh, yeah, 'veak and dizzy.' They *all* say that! We call that 'old Jewish people's VD'. We ignore it."

"Veak and Dizzy" was Mrs. Goldstein's validating symptom. It confirmed to her (and to her significant others—validating symptoms are as much for *others* as for oneself) that she was really sick. Here, in dismissing her "VD," the physician ignored the very first of his patient's presenting symptoms. Whether the woman really felt weak and dizzy doesn't matter. By ignoring that symptom, he tells the patient that "the doctor doesn't care."

Explanatory Models

A key component of all illness is the "explanatory model" or "EM" (see Kleinman 1975 for a thorough discussion). The EM is the patient's explanation for what's going on and includes answers to questions such as

- What do I have?
- What caused it?
- Why me?
- What should be done?
- What will happen if it doesn't get better?

All people, everywhere, have explanatory models for illness. After all, illness (including accidents) is the ultimate cause of death. Illness can maim, disable, distress, inconvenience, or kill; thus, illness threatens everyone. All societies have created medical systems to cope with illness, and explanatory models are central to all medical systems. EMs give meaning to the threatening and potentially terrifying state of being sick. EMs help people organize and manage illness by naming the problem and listing the proper course of action. When an illness has been identified and named, it becomes less intangible and frightening. Resources (both medical and personal) can be mobilized. The illness becomes treatable.

The biomedical accuracy of explanatory models is irrelevant. They are logical to the patient. EMs reflect the patient's everyday experiences. They reflect the meaning of life, health, and misfortune to the patient and his or her family and social network. For example, a white, elderly patient believes that behavioral excesses can cause illness. Liquids too hot or too cold; too much emotion; running or moving too fast—all are "bad for you." She was raised in a neighborhood where her immigrant family were the only members of their ethnic group. Sensitive to instances of ethnic prejudice and desirous of blending into America, the patient's mother insisted that excess of any kind called attention to the family and to their ethnic identity. She was fearful of neighbors pointing to "those kids" who ran too fast, hollered too much, or stood out in any way. "Blend in," she would admonish. "This is America." To this immigrant mother— and to the 100-percent American children she raised—excess was the cause of all things dangerous. That excess should also cause illness is but a logical extension.

Explanatory models are not merely medical curiosities or funky objects for study by anthropologists. As with every other part of an illness, EMs can affect medical management and outcome. The belief (mentioned earlier in our discussion of symptoms) that a pain in the lower left back is "stiffness from working out too hard" reflects the individual's EM. More than being a cute example of culture at work, this explanatory model can keep the sufferer from seeking timely medical care. A study of white, middle-class New York male hypertension patients revealed them to have a common explanatory model that classed nervousness and irritability as symptoms of hypertension (Cohen 1979). These patients' EM further embraced the view that when they subsequently felt "calm" and "in control of themselves," it indicated that their blood pressure was back to normal. Patients with this EM were more likely to become noncompliant by stopping their medications, thus affecting outcome.

The 45-year-old white, middle-class professional man came to the physician practice (owned by the hospital that his HMO contracts with) complaining of a pain in the calf and swelling in his ankle.

The doctor tentatively diagnoses phlebitis. The patient more ten-tatively offers his explanatory model. Being athletic and a regular squash player, he figures his veins are more efficient than those of a less active man. Having larger veins means slower blood flow (log-ically, to him, fluid flows faster through more constricted pipes than through wider pipes). Slower flowing blood is more likely to form a clot than swifter flowing blood. The physician quickly dismisses this EM, and attempts to focus the patient's attention on the "real" causes of blood clots and the potential danger a clot can pose. Here, the doctor's EM stresses pathology and the debili-tating nature of the problem, while the patient's EM stresses the problem's origin in a robust lifestyle and "being too much of a jock." The phlebitis ("an old person's disease," he comments) threatens the patient and his self-image. His EM helps ameliorate the threatening implications. The doctor sees no point in even ne-gotiating an EM.

Here, the patient is left with diminished self-esteem and dimin-ished ownership of the illness. Some trust is lost. The patient may no longer be an active collaborator in treatment.

Explanatory models can range from the mundane ("feed a cold, starve a fever") to the exotic (witchcraft, for example). Kleinman (1980) has noted that the ethnic Chinese EM for mental illness in-volves a perception that mental illness is a condition that disgraces both the sufferer and his or her family. This EM causes many Chinese who suffer emotional distress to avoid demonstrating it or describ-ing clear mental/behavioral symptoms to a physician. Rather, men-tal illness tends to be expressed to the doctor in somatic terms (aches, pains, fatigue, etc.), which are less stigmatizing. A result is confu-sion for the physician and difficulty in diagnosis. Here again, the EM affects care and outcome.

EMs are at the core of all illnesses. Along with their physical symp-toms, patients bring their explanatory models to the physician's of-fice or hospital. EMs are not left at home. By ignoring or minimizing the explanatory model, physicians or nurses tell patients that their beliefs about the problem that threatens their lives, lifestyles, or identities are irrelevant. Biomedicine's EM is more important than the patient's. This is a prescription for dissatisfaction.

Explanatory models, by the way, are a major reason why good explanations and smooth communication are essential in the clinical setting. Precisely because patients *do* present with their own ideas about cause and care, it is necessary to involve them in discussions of diagnosis, treatment, and prognosis. A brief, one-sided, professionally correct statement from the physician, nurse, technologist, or dietician about what's going on may be good for the professional ego but not for effective patient management.

Self-Treatment

With an explanatory model established (albeit only a preliminary one—EMs can evolve as symptoms change or worsen), the next step in the evolution of an illness is, typically, self-treatment. We all do this. It implies that we have made some preliminary diagnosis of our own—and we have. Our EMs direct us to the appropriate remedial action. The student with the possible kidney problem assumes he's just stiff from playing too hard (his EM) and takes some aspirin (the "proper" treatment). Maybe later he'll try some Tylenol with codeine that a roommate or parent has sitting in the medicine cabinet.

Very often, others are brought in for further help with diagnosis and prescribing. Cousin Julia had symptoms similar to yours. It turned out to be such and such and she did so and so for it and it got better, so you take what Julia took. Uncle Ben says your trouble in swallowing is probably a "pulled nerve." You should gargle with salt water twice a day to "neutralize it" and it'll go away, so you try it. None of us rush to seek medical attention unless the symptoms are truly anxiety producing. Hot tea, chicken soup, chamomile, and laxatives—all are common responses to sickness. To this day, my sister is a firm believer that if you have diarrhea and nausea, the best cure is plain rice and an active culture yogurt. But this means that she (like most of us) won't see a doctor until the situation lingers or gets worse. Thus, self-treatment has a significant effect on the disease that is ultimately presented to the physician or brought to the clinical setting for cure.

Ethnicity doesn't really have much effect with regard to the impact of self-treatment on medical care outcome. The herbals or native prescriptions or physical manipulations or prayers or magic of "ethnic" patients merely replace the yogurt or aspirin or teas, soups, and over-the-counter supplements of "nonethnics" as components of self-treatment. From the perspective of the biomedical professional, the result is the same. Self-treatment of any kind may delay "proper" medical treatment and can affect the course of the disease. When I worked at Jackson Memorial Hospital in Miami, we often came across black diabetics who would self-treat before seeing a physician. Their explanatory model for diabetes described it as being "sweet blood." Quite logically, this EM directed sufferers to treat the sweet blood by neutralizing the excess sweetness. Commonly used remedies included infusions of lemon juice or vinegar. Self-treatment here allowed the diabetes to worsen.

The reason self-treatment is so universal is that it typically "works." The vast majority of sicknesses are self-limiting. No matter what you do for it, you eventually recover and give credit to the remedies you used at home or the therapists you visited. Even where the remedies fail, self-treatment strengthens the patient's identification with the illness and his or her responsibility in affecting it. If self-treatment is unsuccessful and the patient must ultimately seek biomedical help, the patient has at least gained some "ownership" over the problem.

In most instances of sickness, the medical professional is the *second* choice and second line of recourse. Self-treatment almost always occurs first. A number of recent surveys indicate that more than 40 percent of Americans may use alternative therapies (herbals, chiropractors, acupuncturists, massage therapists, spiritual healers, etc.) for any given sickness (Cohen 2000; Eisenberg et al. 1998; Reed et al. 1992, 68).

Ethnic group patients may have even more alternate professional resources. Some Puerto Ricans on the East Coast consult *espiritistas*. Miami Cubans may call upon a *santero,* Haitians a *hungan* or voodoo specialist. Some southern Blacks may contact a *root doctor;* Chicago Chinese an *herbalist;* Los Angeles or Denver Mexicans a *curandero.* Trust in formal, mainstream medical providers should not be taken for granted. Numerous reports suggest that Americans spend about as much on alternate therapies as they do on formal medicine. Baby boomers are "into" herbals and supplements at an increasing rate.

The Sick Role

The illness continues to evolve. Symptoms have been identified (some accepted, others rejected as irrelevant), a tentative explanatory model has been applied, and some form of self-treatment has been attempted. The sickness continues and begins to have an effect on the sufferer's activities. At this point, the individual may be admitted to the "sick role." The sick role defines the proper behavior for a sick person and officially identifies the sick person as a "patient" (at this point, a patient of the family, not yet of the physician or hospital). We all have these sick roles. They differ from family to family and ethnic group to ethnic group. Occupancy of the sick role confers certain rights and obligations. For example, if your child is crying and complaining of severe cramps at 7:30 in the morning, you may decide she does not have to go to school. She can stay in bed. You bring her food. You bring her a coloring book. You set up the portable TV on her dresser. She can cry and be irritable and far more demanding than usual and you tolerate it because it's "appropriate." But for these "privileges," she must be compliant (take the medicine you saved from last time, drink all of her tea, etc.), and she can't skip out the door when her friends return from school, with a backward shout of "I'm feeling much better!"

On a more serious level, sick roles define the style of patienthood. Sick roles specify how demanding, complaining, or cooperative the patient should be, also how active or passive in attempting to get well, or, how hopeful or fatalistic in attitude. Explanatory models can affect sick role behavior. The causes patients attribute illness to are "…important precisely because they reveal the meanings patients attach to those symptoms, disabilities, or diseases which they bring to the medical visit. And it is this meaning of illness that determines, in turn, the patient's illness behaviors, coping responses, and emotional reactions" (Stoeckle and Barsky 1981, 225). Thus, the sick role has a clear effect on your ability to manage that patient. Having some idea of the patient's sick role and orientation toward sickness can help you maximize the effectiveness of care provided.

Sick roles develop within families and ethnic groups. If you are sick, you can and should exhibit these behaviors. The expressions of pain by the Italians, Jews, Irish, and Cubans mentioned previously all reflect the content of culturally prescribed and appropriate sick roles. Sick roles are rarely idiosyncratic expressions by patients. Rather, the demanding, complaining, or moaning, the unrealistic cheerfulness, passivity, or denial—all are reflections of behaviors that are regularly rewarded by the patient's family and significant others (they were not invented for the present hospital visit!).

As with explanatory models, sick roles are brought to the hospital along with the medical problem. Of course, medical personnel have their own view of what constitutes a proper sick role for the hospitalized patient. The ideal patient should be compliant, forthcoming with information, collaborative, undemanding, uncomplaining, and appreciative. Patients like this are "good" patients. They make medical management easier and more efficient. Patients who behave otherwise may be labeled as "crocks" or "bad" patients. Lorber's study (1975, 218) of a large New York City hospital demonstrated that nurses and physicians commonly labeled patients as "good" or "problem." "Good" patients were cooperative, uncomplaining, and stoical. Problem patients "made trouble" by complaining, being "over-emotional," and dependent (see also Gordon 1983; Staley 1991). Labels can affect the behavior of those who do the labeling. Staff may take a bit more time in answering when a "bad" patient pushes the call button, or the interaction with a problem patient may be a bit cooler, with more formal professional demeanor and less empathy. Orders for psychological consults may be more likely.

Presenting the Illness to the Doctor

The decision to seek formal medical care is usually a complex one. Symptoms have been discussed with family or friends. Self-treatment is unsuccessful and the patient has reached a threshold level of anxiety, discomfort, or inconvenience. For many, the decision to seek formal medical care is an economic one, where the anxiety or discomfort outweigh the financial implications of seeking formal care. For whatever reason, the medical consult or hospitalization has a certain imperative nature. The patient admits that the problem is beyond the control or realm of knowledge of self and significant others. Performance expectations of the physician or hospital are thus high.

Finally, the sick person stands before the physician. What does the patient tell the professional? Here the patient sifts through everything that has already transpired. Perceived symptoms are selected for presentation that seem appropriate to the situation. Some symptoms may be dropped, others added. As mentioned earlier, Kleinman (1980, 178–220) found that some Chinese mental patients focus on secondary physical complaints, not mentioning psychological problems or symptoms (mental illness being highly stigmatized in Chinese culture).

Physicians often ignore some of the patient's symptoms. The Western disease model of medicine classifies sicknesses into syndromes of co-occurring symptoms. A cold has symptoms of runny nose, sneezing, eye watering, and fatigue (among others), but not symptoms of eye twitching, nervousness, or numbness in the hand. Shingles may itch but not cause the patient to be "veak and dizzy."

Physicians regularly ignore symptoms that do not seem relevant to medically familiar syndromes of disease. Or, once the physician has identified a key medical symptom, secondary symptoms (which can be of great importance to the patient) may be ignored.

For example, a young woman presents to the physician at an outpatient clinic. She complains of pains in both sides of her belly. Suspecting ovarian problems, the doctor's very first response to her symptom presentation is: "When did you have your last period, Miss Smith?" He then asks her about other urogenital problems. Here again, the initial presenting symptom (belly pain) is ignored, telling the patient that her views and sensations are unimportant. In a sense, the doctor has co-opted her problem and turned it into his (not her) disease.

A fascinating ramification of this issue emerged from a study I did in Bogota (Colombia) on patterns of healthcare-seeking by patients who use public medical outpatient clinics and patients who use curanderos (local folk healers). Both groups of patients were similar: largely rural migrants with low-paying blue collar jobs, a low level of formal education, and similar general health problems. When I interviewed both groups of patients, I elicited symptoms by asking "what bothers you" and asking "what else" until no more symptoms were forthcoming. Patients at the folk healer's office listed an average of three or four symptoms. Patients at the outpatient clinic listed an average of six. Why the difference? Further interviews led me to conclude that patients added more symptoms at the clinic to ensure that at least one of the symptoms would be taken seriously and addressed by the physician. The curandero accepted all symptoms, rejecting none and addressing each. By producing more symptoms, the clinic patients were attempting to exert some personal control over the interaction and diagnosis. They anticipated that if they presented only a few symptoms, the doctors might ignore these and create a disease of their own out of the patient's problem, thus co-opting the patient's sickness (Press 1969). Did the clinic patients actually have the additional symptoms? Probably. All of us experience some discomforts in addition to the primary ones we present to our doctors.

Do patients lie to their physicians? Lots of times. Ask any doctor. Patients lie or hide things for many reasons. They may be afraid or ashamed to tell of the "folk" remedies they've already tried. In a fascinating study of physician/patient interaction in the rural south, Murphree and Barrow (1970) noted that in every case they observed, the patient withheld information about use of "old-timey" remedies they had taken prior to seeing the physician. More recently, Eisenberg et al. (1993, 244) finds similar behavior. He notes that "in more than seven of ten instances, users of unconventional therapy did not inform their medical doctor of their use of the therapy."

Patients may also hide symptoms. They may anticipate (and fear) the diagnosis or prognosis and avoid them by minimizing symptoms or severity. Misdirection is not necessarily a conscious ploy. A young medical resident related the following from the outpatient clinic:

> I had an old lady as a patient. She came in complaining of pain at the base of the spine, around the tailbone. I looked and tried everything I could, but wasn't able to diagnose anything. I thought she was goofy. Maybe a month later she came back, this time complaining about pain just below the belly button. I poked and checked, but couldn't find a thing. Then, as part of a routine exam, I gave her a vaginal exam and found a serious infection. On a hunch, I turned her over and checked her anus. Sure enough, she had a significant problem there as well. What I figured was that she viewed doctors as gods and was ashamed to trot out anal or vaginal problems for the 'god' to see. So, she moved the symptoms up out of the 'naughty' areas, to more neutral ground—the tailbone and the area just above the pubic hair line.

When patients omit information about self-treatment, or hide, shift, or reinterpret symptoms, it can affect the course of diagnosis and medical management—as well as the outcome. Thus, such omissions can affect satisfaction with care.

In addition to motives, the language used by patients to present their medical problem can have an effect on the interaction, diagnosis, and treatment. Physicians and nurses prefer articulate patients who can describe things clearly. "Doctor, I have this rather slowly growing pain in my left knee when I try to sleep on my right side, with my knees together. Also, I get a brief stabbing pain whenever I twist my knee to the left." Professionals much prefer this to "Doctor, my leg hurts a lot." Articulate patients with a good vocabulary may be treated with more respect and equality than an inarticulate patient who forces the physician to expend verbal effort in history taking. The physician's explanations and treatment options may be more forthcoming with the "educated" patient than with the less verbal one.

A final, and very important point about illness and the expression of symptoms to medical personnel: when someone—anyone—is sick, physical symptoms are only part of the problems that result. As suggested earlier, sickness can disrupt normal activities and roles. Plans are affected. Self-image is assaulted. This means that every sickness has social and emotional symptoms in addition to the somatic ones. These symptoms are also part of the illness. Patients at the folk healer's office often recite a list of symptoms such as: "Doctor, I have these belly pains, and a constant headache. I'm nervous all the time, and my business is not doing well." The healer accepts all of these as symptoms of a single syndrome. Would a typical physician? Patients in the doctor's office or hospital—whether in Bogota or Peoria—know that physicians and nurses will not take them seriously if they add the non-somatic symptoms they are suffering. Therefore, they fail to mention key factors that affect their well-being and cause anxiety in their daily lives. These disrupted aspects of daily lives are brought with the disease to the clinical setting, and typically go unexpressed and unaddressed.

ROLES AND IDENTITIES

We are the sum total of our roles and identities. Without them we're merely animals. These roles and identities—parent, child, spouse, coworker, neighbor, breadwinner, lover, friend, intellectual, delicate old person, jock, macho, sex pot, cool dude, fox, computer nerd—define who we are. All of these are simultaneously tucked down in our brains and activated as the context and situation requires. Interestingly, one of the few contexts where all or most of our roles and identities are *consciously* present is the hospital. This is because sickness threatens them all. It can make us unattractive. It weakens us and makes us less competent and appealing. When sick we cannot work and provide, or perform domestic tasks appropriately. We become a burden. We cannot meet our obligations to carpool the neighborhood kids (so that our own kids get carpooled in turn). We miss the church meeting we were supposed to attend. Being sick *and* hospitalized takes us out of our normal contexts and makes meeting role obligations impossible.

Threats to roles and self-images accompany every patient and every disease to the hospital. These perceived threats and inconveniences are also part of the illness. Need for a clean room or warm food does not compare with guilt, anxiety, or embarrassment as issues of importance to patients.

On the Press, Ganey inpatient survey we ask patients to rate "staff sensitivity to the problems and inconveniences that sickness and hospitalization can cause." Not surprisingly, this is invariably one of the top three issues most highly correlated with overall satisfaction with care across all hospitals. Treating the patient "like a real person" (a common yet ambiguous phrase) takes on clearer meaning in this context. The "real" person is threatened by having to be in your institution. Thus, effective empathy goes beyond concern for the physical comfort of the patient. Effective empathy must include sensitivity to the person who bears the disease and suffers the illness. When such sensitivity is lacking, the result can be distrust, patient perceptions of staff apathy, or perceived lack of caring attitude on the part of staff. When such sensitivity is present, "it deepen(s) the therapeutic alliance that is at the heart of clinical care" (Levinson et al. 1997).

I remember observing an old lady in an ICU. She had tubes running out of every orifice and she was very sick, but she was conscious. In their ministrations to her, staff repeatedly let her cover sheet slip off. They didn't care because they'd be returning to her with frequency and keeping her naked was more efficient. Anyway, this was an ICU. Staying alive is the key issue—not dignity! The old lady would continuously and feebly reach down to attempt to pull the sheet back over her genital region. This very sick patient was concerned about her dignity and the staff were not. She had brought her identity and personality with her to the ICU. Of course she was aware of and grateful for the heroic care she was receiving; however, the perceived assault to her dignity would likely modify her overall evaluation of this care.

Here's another example from my field notes. I was working with the consultation liaison psychiatry group:

> June 23: We were called up to a medical floor by a young resident. His patient was an eighty-year-old black woman admitted through the ED with suspected congestive heart failure. His repeated attempts to convince her that she needed to have a "blood gas draw" had failed. "Mrs. Jones," he admonished, "we need to draw blood to see how much oxygen is getting to your system. It's important to know this. Now it won't hurt much."
>
> No dice. "Nobody's sticking me!," she insisted. So he called for a psych consult. Up we come and, of course, the first thing she cries out when she sees our psychiatry department ID tags is the expected, "I'm not crazy!" Not surprisingly, she's now even more dissatisfied with care. While the young psych resident was talking with Mrs. Jones, I chatted with her two middle-aged daughters out in the hallway. Had momma ever been to a hospital before? No. Where were her five children delivered, then? At home. Her husband had died several years previously, and since that time she had become the matriarch of a large extended family. She was used to giving orders, not taking them. She assumed responsibility, not dependency. This hospital trip threatened her core identities.
>
> I suggested that the resident try another approach. "Mrs. Jones," he said. "I'm only a resident here. I need to take a blood gas from you or I'll get in trouble. Please let me do it." This worked. Now *she* was back in charge. She agreed to the stick.

But *not* before she had been insulted by the psych consult. Studies indicate that psych consults are very often triggered by poor communication, not inherent psychiatric problems. In many instances the psych consult is a cop-out, an indicator of failure by the medical staff to empathize with and understand the patient. To a significant extent, the barriers to patient compliance and collaboration with the staff lie in the roles and identities threatened by the medical problem, the hospitalization, and the treatment.

THE CLASH OF CULTURES

The evolution of an illness illustrates the complexity of the cultural baggage brought by the patient to the clinical encounter. Symptoms have been sensed and sorted through, some kept, some dropped. Numerous interactions with significant others have confirmed suspicions, named the problem, and tentatively explained it and suggested courses of action. A sick role has been negotiated and legitimated within the family. Self-treatment has been attempted. The decision (typically negotiated with family) to seek formal medical care has been reached. Social, sexual, economic, and other roles have been affected, threatened, or impaired. All of this creates the illness that is brought to the physician or hospital along with any disease. Medical staff, however, are largely trained to recognize and deal with disease. A natural gap exists, and we're talking only about nonethnic, "nonexotic," average American patients with English as their first language who were born and/or raised within the core American popular culture and medical system.

When significant ethnicity enters the picture, it becomes even more complex. "Ethnic" group patients who maintain cultural elements from their country or culture of origin bring additional cultural baggage. Explanatory models become more distanced from common popular notions, as do concepts of healing and appropriate interaction with healthcare professionals. All cultures have their own traditional medical system (regardless of whether Western medicine is "officially" present) and many elements of a different medical system may be maintained by some patients. Language barriers are often but the tip of the iceberg when it comes to establishing understanding, trust, and effective medical management for patients who bring a very different paradigm to the clinical encounter. Cultural as well as linguistic translation may be needed.

CONCLUSIONS

Although much of the preceding discussion is particularly relevant for the physician who must diagnose and devise appropriate treatment for patients, *illness as a cultural construct accompanies every disease to the hospital and to some extent affects every patient's interaction with staff at all levels.* We're not just talking about those staff who deal directly with diagnosing and treating the patient. Every delay, every aspect of body language or tone of voice that could be negatively interpreted, every miscue, every unexplained event or interruption—whether involving transport staff, volunteers, food service, housekeeping, nurses, physicians, or anyone else with whom the patient (and family) comes into contact—tells the patient that his or her problem or concerns are not being taken seriously.

The point of this discussion is to emphasize the complex nature of sickness. Food, amenities, cleanliness, and decor are important infrastructural elements. They certainly play a part in overall satisfaction. So, too (obviously), do technical competence and staff friendliness. But, to paraphrase George Orwell, all patient experiences in the hospital are equal, but some experiences are more equal than others. Patients bring significant cultural baggage—or illness—to the clinical encounter. Satisfaction with care depends to a large extent upon the manner in which staff deal with illness as opposed to the disease, which is clinically defined and technically managed. Not having been to medical or nursing school, patients can only judge clinical quality on the basis of actions and interactions that make sense to them. What makes sense is what addresses things that are

Figure 3.1 Patient Satisfaction (Acute Care Inpatient) Correlated with Likelihood of Recommending Hospital

	Correlation with Likelihood to Recommend
1. How well staff worked together to care for you	0.79
2. Overall cheerfulness of the hospital	0.74
3. Response to concerns/complaints made during your stay	0.68
4. Staff sensitivity to inconvenience that health problems and hospitalization can cause	0.65
5. Amount of attention paid to your special or personal needs	0.65
6. Staff effort to include you in decisions about your treatement	0.63
7. How well the nurses kept you informed	0.63
8. Nurses' attitude toward your requests	0.63
9. Skill of the nurses	0.62
↓	
42. How well things worked (TV, call button, lights, bed, etc.)	0.40
43. Speed of admission process	0.38
44. Temperature of the food (cold foods cold, hot foods hot)	0.37
45. Noise level in and around room	0.37
46. Quality of the food	0.36
47. Room temperature	0.35

Note: n = 1,210,044 patients, 709 hospitals; p = .001; 1/1/99–12/31/99.

Source: Press, Ganey, 2000, "Inpatient Survey." Unpublished.

important to them. Patients understand their illness quite well, even though they may not be able to articulate it in full.

Figure 3.1 ranks all items on the Press, Ganey inpatient survey by their correlation with overall satisfaction. Data were obtained from 1,210,044 patients rating care at 709 hospitals in 2000. A higher correlation coefficient means that the item is more highly linked to overall satisfaction and likely has a stronger "halo effect."

Food and amenities, while still significantly linked with satisfaction, are at the bottom of the list.

Note that the majority of items heading the list reflect illness and interaction rather than technical issues. Coordination of care, inclusion in decision making, information about what's being done, attention to dignity, sensitivity to the personal effect of sickness and hospitalization—these illness-relevant issues have most potential impact on patient satisfaction. The illness/disease distinction is a relevant concern for all who deal with patients, not just physicians.

It must be stressed that to generate patient satisfaction, physicians, nurses, technologists, and others are *not* obliged to cede control of medical management to the patient by acquiescing to any explanatory model or accommodating any behavior or special request for care. Explanations, serious listening, and empathy are key to patient satisfaction—not simply saying "yes" to any patient requests, ideas, and beliefs (Tuckett et al. 1985; Froehlich and Welch 1996).[1]

ACTION FOR SATISFACTION

1. Orient staff to the concept of "patient culture." At the very least, all staff should receive a brief introduction to the concepts of sick role and patient role/identity threats. These aspects of illness have a significant effect on the patient's behavior while in the hospital (that is, on medical management) and are typically expressed in the patient's interaction with a wide range of staff. Chaplains can be great training resources.

2. Respond to patients' symptoms. Listen. Address each symptom, in the order given. Explain why you are focusing on one rather than another of the patient's stated symptoms. This indicates you take the patient seriously and is a key to establishing trust. Many patients

are eager to share their symptoms with others. After all, being sick and hospitalized is a major life event and verbalizing it is cathartic. All personnel should be coached to listen to patients if they want to talk.

3. Identify explanatory models. Attempt to elicit the patient's explanatory model (EM). Try to discern the implications of the EM. Discuss. Never disdain or belittle the patient's EM, but remember its importance to the patient. Explain the biomedical EM in clear language. Make sure the patient understands—a recitation of biomedical jargon won't help. Negotiate the EM if possible to obtain the patient's buy-in to the diagnosis and proposed treatment. Remember that this is not medical school and the patient is not a medical student. If the negotiated EM isn't quite standard medicine, it is not really important, as long as the patient begins to feel at ease with the management program that is appropriate. If the patient does not buy into your EM, dissatisfaction—and non-compliance—are likely to result.

Responding to all symptoms and eliciting the patient's EM is important. When the physician co-opts the patient's problem by imposing the biomedical symptomology and explanatory model, the disease is then "owned" by the physician. This is an important concept for it suggests that if there is any problem (error, complication, comorbidity, poor outcome, etc.), the physician or hospital is at fault because *responsibility* for the disease as well as its cure has been taken from the patient.

4. Understand self-treatment. Elicit what the patient has done for the problem. Everyone self-treats. Get an idea of what the patient thought would work. Don't put down their self-treatment (it might easily reflect long-held family or subcultural traditions that the patient respects). Indicate that the self-treatment reflects a logical response to the patient's EM, thus, the patient does not feel belittled and trust can be established in the biomedical EM and in the

appropriate treatment. Approving of harmless self-treatments the patient appears to favor (and even recommending them when the patient returns home) may encourage trust and compliance with the biomedical regimen.

5. Use patients' sick roles to facilitate medical management. Unless the patient is downright disruptive, work with their behaviors insofar as possible. Remember that the sick role behaviors expressed are likely viewed as appropriate and are rewarded by the patient's family and significant others. These behaviors are not called "roles" for no reason. They are learned and habitual. They provide the patient with a familiar script for expressing anxieties, fears, and needs in the unfamiliar, threatening clinical context. "Retraining" or subtly punishing the patient for "inappropriate" behavior is not the staff's responsibility. Staff must discuss ways in which patient behaviors can be accommodated without judging them to be examples of acting out. "Acting out" is an official negative term describing inappropriate behavior. By labeling patients as acting out, we remove their credibility

6. Acknowledge roles and identities. Staff must be sensitized to the need to elicit patient concerns not only about the course of treatment, but also about the effect of the disease and hospitalization on their lives and perceptions of self. All hospital staff empathize with patients; however, to have an effect, this empathy must be *perceived* by the patient. Hospital staff can easily shift into "clinical mentality." This mode of thinking includes such concepts as those included in the following example.

> Good patients should leave their personal problems at home. They shouldn't bother us by pushing the call button too frequently. They should be compliant, nondemanding, trusting, quiet, and grateful. They should not be concerned with trivia such as personal dignity. After all, they're sick and this *is* a hospital.

This mentality has been responsible all these years for the embarrassing short gowns (an assault to personal dignity), use of first names rather than "Mr." or "Mrs.," labeling of patients "good" and "bad," turfing "problem" patients to psychiatry or social work practitioners, and so forth.

7. Be aware of cultural diversity (ethnicity) as a complicating factor. Staff must have some familiarity with the medical beliefs and expectations of ethnic groups that have a significant representation among your patients. If the interaction between any patient and provider is a cultural transaction, ethnicity obviously complicates it further. Good in-house translators are only the beginning; cultural learning is essential. You may not be able to afford a full-time cultural anthropologist, but you can provide some modest education to your staff on the healthcare beliefs and practices of the major ethnic groups in your patient constituency. If a nearby university has a medical anthropologist on staff, by all means bring him or her in to speak on the medical beliefs of local ethnic groups. You may even wish to bring in a medical anthropologist from outside your area to speak to your staff. You can get a reference from the head of the Society for Medical Anthropology (SMA).[2]

Bring in local ethnic community representatives to talk to your staff. Ideally, get a physician and nurse who are members of the ethnic group(s) to speak. All staff (from top execs to housekeepers and volunteers) must attend. The presenters will likely not be able to give unlimited time and you will want small groups to facilitate discussion, therefore, videotape the presentations. Your translators must attend the presentations and discussions. Shared ethnicity does not mean that all possess the same values and behavioral patterns. Your translators may speak the language, but they may also be second generation and unaware of beliefs and practices common to many in their own ethnic group.

You will need to add relevant materials to your library. Various publications (books and articles) describe health beliefs and practices of ethnic groups (Mexican, Puerto Rican, Laotian, Chinese,

Black American, Native American, Haitian, etc.). Several journals focus on diversity in healthcare. Among them are *Holistic Nursing Practice, Journal of Cultural Diversity,* and the *Journal of Multicultural Nursing and Health.* Some good general references include:

- Spicer's (1977) *Ethnic Medicine in the Southwest;*
- Alan Harwood's (1981) edited volume *Ethnicity and Medical Care;*
- Galanti's (1991) *Caring for Patients from Different Cultures;*
- Spector's (1991) *Cultural Diversity in Health and Illness;*
- Dobson's (1991) *Transcultural Nursing;*
- Giger and Davidhizar's (1995) *Transcultural Nursing: Assessment and Intervention;*
- Andrews and Boyle's (1995) *Transcultural Concepts in Nursing Care;*
- Lipson et al.'s (1996) *Culture and Nursing Care: A Pocket Guide;* and
- Purnell and Paulanka's (1998) *Transcultural Health Care: A Culturally Competent Approach.*

NOTES

1. Physicians may find it quite useful to review Platt's discussions (1992; 1995) of good and bad doctor/patient communication. His verbatim examples of history-taking illustrate many of the principles discussed in this chapter, and the potential therapeutic consequences of (not) understanding "where the patient's coming from."

2. As the office and leadership of the SMA changes annually, get in touch with the parent American Anthropological Association (AAA) for the name of a contact in the SMA. AAA offices are at 4350 N. Fairfax Dr., Suite 640, Arlington, VA 22203, or www.aaanet.org.

REFERENCES

Andrews, M., and J. S. Boyle (eds.). 1995. *Transcultural Concepts in Nursing Care.* Philadelphia: Lippincott.

Cohen, J. 2000. "Reckoning with Alternative Medicine." *Academic Medicine* 75: 571.

Cohen, L. 1979: "Culture, Disease and Stress Among Latino Immigrants." Special Study R11ES. Washington, D.C.: Smithsonian Institution.

Dobson, S. M. 1991. *Transcultural Nursing*. London: Scutari Press.

Eisenberg, D., R. Kessler, C. Foster, F. Norlock, D. Calkins, and T. Delbanco. 1993. "Unconventional Medicine in the United States." *New England Journal of Medicine* 328: 246-52.

Eisenberg, D. 1977. "Diseases and Illness." *Culture, Medicine and Psychiatry* 1: 9-23.

Eisenberg, D., R. Davis, S. Ettner, S. Appel, S. Wilkey, M. Van Rompay, and R. Kessler. 1998. "Trends in Alternative Medicine Use in the United States, 1990-1997: Results of a Follow-up National Survey." *JAMA* 280: 1569-75.

Froehlich, G., and H. Welch. 1996. ""Meeting Walk-in Patients' Expectations for Testing: Effects on Satisfaction." *Journal of General Internal Medicine* 11: 470-74.

Galanti, G.-A. 1991. *Caring for Patients from Different Cultures: Case Studies from American Hospitals*. Philadelphia: University of Pennsylvania Press.

Giger, J., and R. Davidhizar (eds). 1995. *Transcultural Nursing: Assessment and Intervention*. St. Louis: Mosby Year Book.

Gordon, D. 1983. "Hospital Slang for Patients: Cracks, Gomers, Gorks, and Others." *Language in Society* 12 (2): 173-85.

Harwood, A. (ed). 1981. *Ethnicity and Medical Care*. Cambridge, MA: Harvard University Press.

Hautman, M. A., and J. Kreider Harrison. 1982. "Health Beliefs and Practices in Middle-Income Anglo-American Neighborhood. *Advances in Nursing Science* 5 (Apr): 49-64.

Kleinman, A. 1975. "Explanatory Models in Health Care Relationships." *In Health and the Family (National Council for International Health Symposium)*. NCIH159-172.Washington, D.C.

Kleinman, A., L. Eisenberg, and B. Good. 1978. "Clinical Lessons from Anthro-pologic and Cross-Cultural Research." *Annals of Internal Medicine* 88: 251-58.

Kleinman, A. 1980. *Patients and Healers in the Context of Culture*. Berkeley, CA: University of California Press.

Lambert, W., E. Libman, and E. Poser. 1960. "The Effect of Increased Salience of a Membership." 38: 350-57.

Lipson, J., S. Dibble, and P. Minarik. 1996. *Culture and Nursing Care: A Pocket Guide.* San Francisco: University of California at San Francisco Press.

Lorber, J. 1975. "Good Patients and Problem Patients: Conformity and Deviance in A General Hospital." *Journal of Health and Social Behavior* 16: 213-25.

Levinson, W., D. Roter, J. Mullooly, V. Dull, and R. Frankel. 1997. "Physician-Patient Communication: The Relationship with Malpractice Claims Among Primary Care Physicians and Surgeons." *JAMA* 277 (7): 553-59.

Murphree, A., and M. Barrow. 1970. "Physician Dependence, Self-Treatment Practices and Folk Remedies in a Rural Area." *Southern Medical Journal* 63: 403-408.

Platt, F. 1995. *Conversation Repair: Case Studies in Doctor-Patient Communication.* Boston: Little, Brown.

Platt, F. 1992. *Conversation Failure.* Tacoma, WA: Life-Sciences Press.

Press, I. 1969. "Urban Illness: Physicians, Curers, and Dual Use in Bogota." *Journal of Health and Social Behavior* 10: 209-18.

Purnell, L., and B. Paulanka. 1998. *Transcultural Health Care: A Culturally Competent Approach.* Philadelphia: F.A. Davis.

Reed, J. C. 1992. "Alternative Systems of Medical Practice." *Alternative Medicine: Expanding Medical Horizons.* Washington, D.C.: U.S. Department of Health.

Spector, R. 1991. *Cultural Diversity in Health and Illness.* Norwalk, CT: Appleton and Lange.

Spicer, E. H. 1977. *Ethnic Medicine in the Southwest.* Tucson, AZ: University of Arizona Press.

Staley, J. 1991. "Physicians and the Difficult Patient." *Social Work* 36 (1): 74-79.

Stoeckle, J., and A. Barsky. 1981. "Attributions: Uses of Social Science Knowledge in the 'Doctoring' of Primary Care." In *The Relevance of Social Science for Medicine,* edited by L. Eisenberg and A. Kleinman, 223-40. Dudrecht, Holland: D. Reidel.

Tuckett, D., M. Boutlon, C. Olson, and A. Williams. 1985. *Meetings Between Experts: An Approach to Sharing Ideas in Medical Consultations.* London: Tavistock.

Zborowski, M. 1952. "Cultural Components in Responses to Pain." *Journal of Social Issues* 8 (4): 16-30.

Zola, I. K. 1966. "Culture and Symptoms: An Analysis of Patients' Presenting Complaints." *American Sociological Review* 31: 615-30.

CHAPTER 4

From Theory to Method

Patient satisfaction measurement is *not* typical market research; therefore, proper methodology is extremely important. You're probably already measuring patient satisfaction, and we established the rationale for it in the first chapter. In this chapter, we are concerned with making sure you're doing it right.

REPORT CARDS VS. QUALITY IMPROVEMENT INSTRUMENTS

Because patient satisfaction is important, it has to be monitored, and others besides yourself will be monitoring your patients' satisfaction. You will be held accountable for patient satisfaction; are you measuring it properly? An increasing number of state hospital associations are making public the results of sporadic surveys being sent to the patients of member institutions. Business/purchasing coalitions have done the same (and use the data to influence contracts with providers).

These "report cards" will increase in frequency. Various outside entities may be measuring (or requiring you to measure for them) your patients' satisfaction. Their measurement tools will be serving someone else's agenda—not yours.

Report Cards Are Emphatically Not QI Instruments

Report cards and QI instruments have very different functions. Surveys for report cards are typically conducted annually. They provide sporadic snapshots. Their function is accountability, not improvement. Data may be reported by DRG or procedure, but are not usually broken out by nursing unit, physician, and so forth. Nor should they be. Report cards are for outside evaluation of your general institutional quality. You will be held accountable for the scores, but report cards usually won't give you sufficient information with which to address bad numbers. Report cards cannot provide the kinds of information you need to identify specific problems or high performers and to design specific initiatives for quality improvement. Certainly report cards cannot help you monitor quality. Monitoring is an ongoing, not sporadic activity.

I don't want anyone confusing two very different kinds of instruments and functions. An administrator who relies solely on someone else's report card to sporadically monitor patient satisfaction will not achieve the institution's goals or live its mission. Regardless of whether you send out surveys for a report card (required by a state hospital association, for example), you must also send out surveys on a continuing basis for quality improvement purposes. You cannot address issues raised by a report card without detailed in-house information collected on a regular basis.

POSSIBILITIES AND LIMITATIONS OF SATISFACTION SURVEYS

If you have got to measure patient satisfaction, the data can be remarkably useful. You will have satisfaction scores for all of your major service sectors (inpatient, ED, ambulatory surgery, home health, etc.). You will be able to monitor satisfaction by nursing units, departments, medical specialties, doctors, payers, technologists—and just about anyone or anything else whose performance and effect on patients you want to monitor. But don't let anyone fool you by claiming that satisfaction survey data will solve your problems by themselves—they can't. Survey data are limited by the number of questions you want to ask. Ask too few and you won't get sufficient information; ask too many and you cut the return rate substantially.

Each patient in your institution experiences thousands of interactions with your people, equipment, and physical plant. You cannot ask questions about each experience. Take admitting, for example. You could easily ask about chair comfort, privacy, courtesy, friendliness (quite different from courtesy), knowledge, speed, accuracy, and redundancy ("Did we ask you the same domestic and financial questions while registering this time that we asked you the last time you were here?"). You could ask about lighting, lobby noise, introductions, explanations, directions to rooms, and expression of concern. You could ask 20 more questions about admitting alone, but by that time the patient will have tossed the survey into the garbage can.

The surveys cannot identify root causes of problems. Let's say you get low scores on "courtesy of the person who admitted you." This is an important issue. But can you identify its underlying cause? As we noted, you cannot ask everything. Perhaps the low courtesy score is caused by a high census. Perhaps the admitting clerk is forced to answer phones and can't pay continuous attention to the people being admitted. Perhaps the physical layout of the admitting desk makes it appear "bank lobby-like" and too impersonal or intimidating. Perhaps the admitting clerk is new and unsure. Perhaps the clerk has an attitude toward Medicaid or certain minority patients.

You cannot ask patients everything; even if you could, their answers still would not necessarily reveal underlying cause. A low score on "nurse's response to the call button," might have any number of possible causes—none of which are obvious to the patient. Is the problem the call light location and visibility in the nursing station? A high census? Understaffing? Mechanical failure? (Maybe the call button is designed in such as way as to prevent electrical contact when pressed in a particular manner. All the patient knows is that she has pushed it and no one responds.) Is it callous nurses? Is it pesky, demanding patients (who have been labeled and are being "punished" by nurses who wait just a bit longer before responding to the call)? Here again, a low score tells you only that you have a particular problem—It is up to you to dig deeper into the issue to discover the underlying cause. No survey can do more than identify the existence and intensity of a problem. Staff have to follow through with cause identification and problem-solving techniques.

WHAT ARE PATIENT SATISFACTION SURVEYS REALLY MEASURING?

Satisfaction surveys capture patients' recollections and perceptions of care. "Recollections" and "perceptions" may not necessarily correspond with events as they "actually" happened. In a large sense, the issue of "reality" is quite unimportant. With patient satisfaction, reality is in the eye of the patient, not the person writing or reading the survey.

Even if the patient is asked an outright question about whether an event occurred (answerable by "yes" or "no"), the response reflects a subjective recollection, not necessarily reality. I recall a colleague reporting on a study of informed consent at a hospital. The interactions between surgeons and their patients were videotaped. Following surgery and recovery, patients were asked whether they had been given information about the procedure and potentially negative outcomes. Many patients who claimed *not* to have been given information prior to surgery actually had received such information. The researchers concluded that it was the quality of the interaction (friendliness, receptivity to questions, not appearing rushed) with the physician that governed the quantity of technical information remembered.

If a simple yes/no question can yield subjective responses, questions offering a scale of answers provides even more opportunity for subjective judgement by the patient. "How many minutes did you wait for the doctor?" asks one survey. If the patient circles the "10 minutes" response, is it the case that the doctor actually arrived within 10 minutes, or did it "just seem like it" to the patient? If the patient is given a choice of five possible responses (never, almost never, sometimes, usually, always) to the question "How often did the nurse respond within 5 minutes of your pushing the call button?," what is being elicited are perceptions, impressions, and evaluations—not an account of real events. Nurses could always respond to the call button within 5 minutes and you'd still have a full range of responses to the "how often..." question. A patient who was in pain, or anxious, or frightened, bored, impatient, or cantankerous might respond with "never." A patient who was well-informed, comfortable, and had trust in the staff might respond with "always," even though response time might have been as high as 15 minutes.

Again (and I cannot stress this enough), if you have a low score for response time to the call button, this doesn't necessarily mean you have a time problem. It could easily (more easily) be a communication problem.

Patient satisfaction is indeed subjective. If someone promises you that their survey gets at what "really" happens in your hospital, don't believe it. All surveys tap perceptions (call them "impressions" or "ratings" or whatever you wish), not objective reality. These perceptions create the patient's reality. As the whole goal of patient satisfaction measurement is to elicit the patient's evaluation of care, not the provider's—the issue of "accuracy" is irrelevant. If patients think a wait is too long, a room too blah, a shot too painful, an explanation too obtuse, it is. Are you going to say, "Hey, these patients are nuts! Ignore them!"? Regardless of their accuracy, you have to address these issues or your patients will continue to be dissatisfied and disloyal. If survey results show that your patients are dissatisfied, you have a very real problem.

DOS AND DON'TS OF PATIENT SATISFACTION MEASUREMENT

Patient satisfaction measurement is emphatically not your usual market research. Remember, these customers would much rather *not* be using your services! Second, patients are intimidated by modern medicine and hospitals. Airline or hotel or auto dealers' customers are not intimidated by their providers. By and large, patients are reluctant to criticize doctors, nurses, or hospitals. They don't want to bite the hand that heals them. Thus, the real problem in measuring patient satisfaction is getting patients to criticize—not compliment. Reflecting this, on most hospitals' surveys with a 5-point answer scale, 90 percent of patients rate hospital care at 4 or 5—the two top response categories.

Because patients are reluctant to criticize, you must minimize the potential for biasing their responses toward the positive. Survey design is a science. A lot is known about ways in which respondents are potentially biased. Following are guidelines for your patient survey methods.

Use Mail-back Surveys Rather than Telephone Surveys

Because patients are intimidated by healthcare, their "cover is blown" when they are phoned at home. They are no longer anonymous, but are being interviewed by a representative of the provider, who will "tell" on them. The patient may have to use this provider again in the near future. In several studies conducted on the relative advantages of phone versus mail-back patient surveys, phone surveys were found to yield higher scores. This is because patients are reluctant to criticize the provider in person, on the phone.

Phoned patients tend to move their responses up to a higher category so as not to offend the caller, thus respondents give fewer lower marks. This "acquiescence bias" is a key feature of phone patient satisfaction surveys (Hall 1995; Ware 1995). Now, even with the mail-back method, patients may assume that the provider will be able to identify them via a bar code or other complex number on the survey. Nonetheless, the patient fills it out in the privacy of home and need not provide a written name. At least the possibility of anonymity exists.

Another disadvantage of phone surveys is that respondents cannot see the answer scale, and so this must be continuously repeated. Confusion could result. Patients may also grow bored with the questioning (and intrusion on their TV, dinner, or leisure time) and give all "5s," just to speed things up.

Speaking of speeding things up, some phone survey companies may require interviewers to probe and ask patients for explanations if they give a low satisfaction response (a 1, 2, or 3, for example). Respondents quickly learn that if they stop giving negative responses they'll speed up the interview.

Because of the intimidation and interruption factors, phone surveys cannot elicit as many comments as can written surveys. The very fact that someone is on the other end of the line awaiting a response can create a "hurry-up" atmosphere that discourages comments—particularly thoughtful ones.

Phone surveys are far more costly, compared with the same number of responses obtained through the mail method.

Don't let anyone fool you about response rates to phone surveys of patient satisfaction. Some firms claim to get 60 percent or higher response. 60 percent of what? Certainly not of your total patient population. Given the high cost of phone surveys, only a small sample of total discharges are called. How many of them don't have phones? Are not home when called? Refuse to answer when called? What phone surveyors usually mean (and usually do not publicize) when they claim a 60-percent response rate, is that 60 percent of those who actually answer the phone may agree to be surveyed. This *net* response rate could be quite a small percentage of your total patient population.

Finally, what do *you* do when you get a telemarketing call in the evening? How often do you interrupt your dinner or leisure time TV to answer a survey? What with caller ID, phone programs that block calls from unknown numbers, and state regulations permitting phone owners to ban telemarketing calls, telemarketing will likely disappear or be severely constricted in the near future. Under these circumstances, will those who actually answer phone surveys be representative of your customer population?

For all these reasons, Don Dillman (who wrote the "bible" of survey research: *Mail and Telephone Surveys,* first edition, 1978) recently concluded that phone surveys were no longer practical. "It is becoming more difficult than in the past to complete telephone surveys" (Dillman 2000, 8).

Recognize the Differences Between Internet, Hand-out, and Real-time Surveys

Surveying patients via the Internet may not be a viable alternative to the mails. Most patients, including the elderly and low-income patients, have addresses, even phones, but not computers and e-mail. Many are not at ease with computer use. Thus, patients who can and will respond to an Internet survey automatically represent a biased sample. If Internet-surveyed patients are required to log onto a hospital's website, the effort may cut response rates significantly. If patients are surveyed via email, their anonymity is automatically compromised.

Surveying patients while they are still in the hospital or medical office raises additional issues of potential bias. Patients are intimidated by healthcare providers and are generally reluctant to criticize the hand that heals them—particularly if that hand is still actively involved in their care!

"Real time" surveying implies that you collect patient evaluations while they are still in-house and then analyze the information—and respond to it—on the spot. This can be done several ways:

1. Hand the survey to the patient; collect it afterward.
2. Provide the patient with a small, hand-held computing device that shows the questions and has five buttons for the answer scale.
3. Broadcast the survey on an in-house TV channel and again provide the patient with a response device.
4. Use an "IVR" (interactive voice response) method wherein the patient dials a certain number on the bedside phone and is verbally led through a prerecorded survey that requires touching a number on the phone to respond.

The paper survey must be scanned or the data entered for analysis. The other three methods involve automatic computer analysis to derive mean scores as each patient completes the survey.

The problem with analysis of real-time data is the very small number of daily surveys; you might be tempted to overreact to negative responses. But a more serious problem is potential whitewash. While patients are still under your control (especially while they are still in your bed!) the potential for intimidation is great and you are unlikely to get many criticisms. You want realistic information, not falsely positive numbers. Real-time patient satisfaction measurement sounds enticing, but may not provide the kind of useful information you want.

Do Not Include Photos of Kindly Staff or Satisfied Patients

You are trying to get information, not influence potential customers; the survey is emphatically not a marketing tool. The goal is to make the appearance and "feel" of the survey as neutral as possible so as not to affect responses. As I indicated earlier, patients lean toward not biting the hand that heals them. So include no glowing mission statements and no photos of kindly staff, hovering over grateful patients. These essentially tell patients to give you a good score, and they will be inclined to comply.

Encourage Mail Back and Honesty in the Cover Letter Accompanying the Survey

If your cover letter waxes eloquent about the amazing quality of your institution, this could discourage the patient from filling out the survey. Why should the patient bother if you already know you're high quality? Or, if the patient does fill out the survey, the strongly positive cover letter may bias the response. Tell the patient that it's okay to complain about something. Survey cover letter writing is a science. An effective letter has the following characteristics:

1. A very minimal statement about the provider's *desire* to be a quality institution.
2. A brief statement of what is wanted.
3. A request for negative, as well as positive evaluations.
4. A "reward" for the patient—ideally a compliment (that is, a statement that reflects the patient's importance to the quality improvement process).
5. The letter is very short, with short sentences and paragraphs.

Various tangible rewards can be offered to patients to complete and mail back the survey. Enclose a movie or fast-food coupon, for example. One hospital encloses a drawing coupon with each survey. If returned with the survey, the coupon goes into a monthly drawing that offers $25 gift certificates (typically for a fast-food restaurant) to winners. The hospital claims that return rates have increased by 5 percent since the drawing was initiated.

Figure 4.1 Survey Cover Letter

Dear Mrs. Xxxxx,

You were recently treated at Central General Hospital. We want to provide the very best care for you and your family. But to do so, we need to know what we're doing right and what needs improvement. We depend on our patients to give us this important information.

We need your help!

Please fill out the enclosed survey as honestly as possible, and send it back in the enclosed envelope. We promise we'll pay attention.

Many thanks,
Joe Administrator

An ideal cover letter is on a separate sheet of paper, not printed on the survey itself. If possible, use the patient's name. Figure 4.1 illustrates a possible cover letter; notice how short it is.

Group the Questions in Logical Sections that Capture Important Linked Experiences

By grouping questions, you are more likely to receive feedback about specific areas of care. For example, you may wish to ask questions about preadmission testing, and you certainly need to ask some questions about admitting. You should also ask patients to rate your food, amenities, and housekeeping. Obviously you need a section on nursing. As patients' evaluation of care is inevitably influenced by relatives and friends who may have visited and interacted with staff, a complete survey must also ask about the experiences of visitors and family. Lab and radiology experiences are shared by many patients and these, too, should constitute a section of the survey. Discharge is obviously important (instructions, efficiency, continuity of care issues) and requires a separate section near or at the end of the survey. Finally, ask how well physicians interacted with and cared for patients. These could include either staff physicians (for a teaching hospital) or outside attendings. Make sure you specify which you mean.

Include Food and Housekeeping Questions

For anyone who asks if it's necessary to include questions about food and amenities in an ostensibly "quality of care"–oriented survey, the answer is emphatically, "Yes!" Room, housekeeping, and food are issues all patients can empathize with, understand, and evaluate. For bored or disoriented patients, meals mark the times of the day. They are activity high points. The room and amenities surround the patient 24 hours a day, affecting interaction and mood. Patients who view the food as bad and the room and cleanliness as substandard are less likely to feel they have had the best of care overall. While we find that food and room scores are far less highly correlated with overall satisfaction, the correlation coefficients are still at .4 and above. This means they are indeed linked to overall satisfaction, just not as highly as nursing or other aspects of care.

Put food and housekeeping questions near the beginning of the survey, before nursing and physician items. Remember the issue of intimidation, and the importance of getting patients to respond as honestly as possible. Ask patients to rate more neutral items before asking them to evaluate more "sensitive" elements of care (nursing, physicians, etc.). If you do have some problems with nursing, physicians, or technologists, you are more likely to coax realistic evaluations out of patients once they've already assigned a lower score or two for some neutral item such as "temperature of the food" or "daily cleaning of the room." Note: Just because patients give a low score to food or room issues does not imply that they will therefore give nursing low scores. If your nursing is great, you'll get a lot of "5s" regardless of low food scores!

Write the Questions from the Patients' Perspective so that the Questions Reflect Their Level of Knowledge, Not the Organization's

Do not use words like "advance directives" or "attending physician." Patients may not know the difference between an in-house attending physician and their own private doctor. "Doctor" is a better word than "physician." Use "ER" rather than "emergency department." Do not ask about student nurses, LPNs, nurses' assistants, physician assistants, residents or any other subcategories of staff that patients could confuse with senior professionals. Patients typically will remember only that there were doctors, nurses, and specific types of therapists (respiratory, occupational). They will probably remember the person who served them food, cleaned their rooms, and attended to their spiritual needs. They may remember the admitting clerk. They will probably remember which gizmos (bed, TV) worked and which did not.

The wording in the survey should not exceed the sixth-grade level.

Use Only One Answer Scale

You might be tempted to use different answer scales for different sections of your survey. Don't. Patients will get confused. Moreover, if the responses to some questions are "yes" and "no," to others "agree" or "disagree," to others "very poor" to "very good," and to yet others "always" to "never," you will not be able to compare sections easily or derive a single performance score for the whole institution. Use a single answer scale throughout the entire survey.

THE NUMBER OF RESPONDENTS

You need a sufficient number of respondents for several reasons. First, and most important, you want statistically valid numbers.

Always be cognizant of the number of respondents that generate your data. When small numbers of patients respond, scores can jump around from period to period and not reflect statistically significant changes. A small nursing unit might generate only a half dozen responses during the monitoring period. A few patients who are unusually negative or positive can affect unit scores dramatically; but the variation is not statistically significant and is probably not representative of the unit's general quality. The same thing goes for emergency department surveys that identify individual physicians. The mean score generated by a handful of surveys should not be used for serious performance evaluation. To rely on such small numbers for QI initiatives may do more harm than good. Never over-react (either positively or negatively) to scores based on low numbers of returns. This is where *trending* comes in. Monitoring your numbers over time can show trends that reflect growing care problems—or growing care successes. If units with a small "n" (the number of returned surveys) sustain their scores or continue period after period in the same upward or downward direction, the data can be viewed as a trend, taken seriously, and should generate an appropriate response. The key is not to overreact to one-time satisfaction scores of units, departments, or staff with few survey respondents. This, by the way, is another reason not to rely on one-shot or annual "report cards" for your ongoing quality improvement and performance-recognition programs.

Another reason for wanting more respondents is that it allows you to go deeper into the data, breaking it down by different characteristics (and have sufficient respondents in each category to offer statistically significant results). For example, if you wanted to look at quality of IV starts by nursing unit *and* break the scores down by age within each unit, you obviously need a higher number of survey returns per unit. If you get 10 returns for a nursing unit you might wind up with 2 or 3 patients in each age category, which is essentially useless information (or even dangerous information, if precipitous action is taken based on these few returns). A minimum "n" of 30 to 50 per inpatient unit can facilitate this kind of analysis. A minimum of 100 per shift will work for the emergency department, although more returns allow more types of data breakdowns.

WHAT ABOUT SAMPLING AND RESPONSE RATES?

You want the data to be statistically significant. Simple sampling can do this. The ideal sampling would be to send a survey to every discharged patient. Such a mailing is great PR, as it tells every patient that you are interested in his or her evaluation of care and want to do something about it. Compare the demographics (percent of each age, sex, length of stay, first-timer or repeat visit, etc.) of those who return the survey with the demographics of your whole hospital population. If you are mailing to all or sampling a significant portion of your discharges, respondent demographics should closely approximate your patient population.

If you do not want to send a survey to all of your inpatients, send one to half (mailing to every other discharged patient). You will probably want to sample less than 100 percent of your ED patients because the numbers are high and the costs of mailing and handling can be significant.

Typically, a single-wave mailing (cover letter and survey) will yield anywhere from 25 to 35 percent response to a well-designed inpatient survey and cover letter. Hospitals in larger cities might get a somewhat lower response rate. Smaller, more rural institutions get higher return rates. If you send a two-wave mailing, you are typically adding a reminder postcard one week or ten days after the initial survey goes out. Our research indicates that response rates are boosted by only 3 or 4 percentage points by sending a reminder postcard. The reason for the low additional response is that by the time the patient has been home for a couple of weeks, the original survey has usually been trashed. At the time of this writing, the effect of HIPAA privacy regulations on open postcards to ex-patients is still unclear. An outright ban is possible. So, overall, forget the postcard (even if you use a folded, closed type of card). Too little is gained for the added cost and effort.

A three-wave mailing typically adds another copy of the survey a week or ten days after the postcard. This can increase response rates to 40 or 45 percent, but also adds to the cost. You can save on some printing and postage by tracking returns (via a patient identifier on each survey and/or return envelope) and removing these patients from the second and third mailing lists. This obviously complicates the process. Is such complication necessary?

In the experience of Press, Ganey, multiple mailings do not result in data that differ significantly from data that you can obtain with a single survey mail-out. (Obviously, I personally prefer that my hospital clients do multiple mailings because it increases my company's profit!)

We have found that a single mailing and a 25 to 30 percent return rate yields very stable, reliable scores and statistically significant data. It's the *number* of returns you get, not the *percent* return rate that determines the validity of your data. You can phone 20 people and get responses from 10 of them. That's a response rate of 50 percent—but the validity of the data is affected by the mere 10 respondents. If you are measuring patient satisfaction in your ED and using random sampling techniques, you are better off getting 100 responses per shift (representing only a 20 percent return rate) than 30 per shift representing a 60 percent return rate.

THE ISSUE OF "RESPONSE BIAS"

Let's be realistic about "response rates." No magic response rate (say, 50 percent) guarantees validity. What is important is that the type of respondents stays relatively consistent and representative. If the patients who respond to your survey are consistent in terms of gender (percent females and males), age (percent between 50 and 60 years of age, etc.), and procedures (percent surgical or medical patients, etc.), the survey results should be reliable even if the response rate is only 10 percent (assuming the number of respondents is sufficient).

Even if the demographics of respondents don't perfectly match your hospital patient population, survey results are useful so long as the respondent "bias" remains consistent. For example, assume that your patient population is split evenly between males and females, and that patients who respond to your survey include 60 percent female and 40 percent male. Let's say that this biased sample gives you a score of 85 for a particular survey item. Assume further that if the respondents had been evenly split between males and females, the score would have been 83. Does it matter that your score should "really" be 83, not 85? The answer is no, it doesn't matter—as long as your returned surveys continue to reflect a consistent bias of 60 percent females. The reason the bias does not matter is that the survey scores—83 or 85 or 79—are not meaningful or important in themselves. The scores signal change or stability in your performance. Thus, if you improve staff performance on the item in question, it might go up by 3 points (from 83 to 86). If your base were 85, it would still go up 3 points (to 88) if you improved performance. Either way, the score moves. Whether the score is 83, 85, or 79, doesn't matter. If the composition of the patients returning the survey remains constant and if your performance on that particular item remains constant, the score will remain constant as well. Similarly, if you change your performance, the scores should change. A 3-point decrease or increase is a real 3-point decrease or increase. This, and not the number in itself, is what counts. In sum, don't get hung up on response rates, but monitor the demographics of respondents to make sure their composition is consistent.

THE ISSUE OF "NONRESPONSE BIAS"

So, who is returning the surveys? The whackos and those with an axe to grind? What about the 60 or 70 percent of patients who don't respond to the survey? Could they have a totally different view of your quality of care? It is not likely. As we have already indicated, (a) increasing the response rate through multiple-wave mailings does not change the data significantly, and (b) the vast majority of patients responding to a first mailing rate care as "4" or "5" (the top two response categories). Moreover, we find that with a single mailing and 20 to 30 percent return rate, respondents' demographics (age, gender, etc.) are representative of your patient population.

A problem with using multiple-wave mailings to increase response rate is that those who don't respond until the second and third waves are filling the survey out many weeks after discharge. They remember less about their care and can only respond with general impressions rather than specific recollections of events and interactions. Maybe they have received their bills by then; maybe they (unrealistically) feel they should be healing and getting back to normal activities faster. With each passing week after discharge, additional life events can have an effect on recollections and evaluations of care during the hospitalization. That is why I feel that a single-wave mailing sent out within a day or two of discharge offers the most reliable, accurate, consistent, cost-effective, and useful information.

MAXIMIZING RETURN RATES

Regardless of how many you send out, you want the maximum number of returns. Here are some suggestions:

1. Make sure your cover letter is appropriate (refer back to the previous discussion) and that your survey is not too long.
2. Do not over-survey patients, this cuts return rates. Many patients get pre-admit testing in the outpatient setting before coming to inpatient. They can receive both inpatient and outpatient surveys if you aren't careful. If the problem started with an ED visit, the patient might get a third survey. Here,

the department managing your survey (whether sending them out or providing names and addresses to an outside contractor) has to have good discharge data so as to prevent multiple surveying.

3. Send the surveys out as soon as possible after discharge. The quicker the patient gets the survey, the more likely it will be filled out. The event is still fresh and patients are still anxious to rehash it. After a couple of weeks, patients have told everyone they know about their sickness and hospitalization. It's getting to be old news and the patient is getting bored talking (or writing) about it. Surveys mailed to patients months after discharge yield data of little utility. Specific events and staff will have been forgotten.

4. Make sure patients know about the survey before they leave the hospital. Prepare them to expect a survey shortly after they get home. Tell them how important it is to you. Holy Cross Hospital in Chicago scripts this. Staff are encouraged to say the following to patients (or paraphrase it) while they are still in the hospital:

Customer satisfaction is very important to all of us at Holy Cross. We're committed to serve you. After you're discharged you'll receive a survey in the mail. It's important to us to know what's pleased you and what's fallen short of your expectations. We ask that when you receive the survey, you complete it and mail it back. If there is anything during your stay that we could solve right now, please let us know.

Staff are required to inform patients about the survey both at admission and at discharge.

A laminated copy of the survey is displayed to patients. I have seen copies of Holy Cross' survey taped to the ceiling above an x-ray table, with the lab/x-ray section circled! In addition, the hospital implemented a monthly contest in which the nursing unit with the highest percentage of returned surveys wins a pizza party.

For general encouragement of patients, Holy Cross also has given coupons for free cholesterol screening to patients who return the survey. Moreover, a reminder about the survey appears on the discharge instruction form given patients prior to leaving the hospital.

All of these maneuvers can improve return rates. Holy Cross claims that promoting the survey prior to discharge boosted survey returns by 10 percent.

Brown County General in Georgetown, Ohio hands out a pen to discharged patients with the message "Your opinion counts." A sticker on the patient's discharge instructions reminds them that a survey will be coming. Brown County also found that follow-up phone calls to patients reminding them to fill out their surveys increased response rates by fully 10 to 20 percent.

While it might be thought that making reminder calls is not cost effective, the reminder can—and should—be tagged on to a much more important message. Columbus Regional (Indiana) phones every inpatient after discharge, to see how they are doing and if they have any questions. This call is a powerful demonstration of caring and a brief reminder about the survey adds little time or cost to it.

ENCOURAGING WRITTEN COMMENTS ON THE SURVEYS

You will want lots of written comments. Survey questions themselves cannot identify root causes of problems; you get at these through the comments patients write. You don't just want praise and lavishly positive statements that you can use in your marketing. Even more important is receiving information about what's *not* working. You can encourage more honest comments by asking for them:

COMMENTS (please describe good or bad experiences)

By asking for "bad" experiences as well as "good," you tell patients that it's okay to complain. Many healthcare professionals are loathe to suggest to patients that they might have been dissatisfied with anything. Asking for "suggestions for improvement" pussyfoots around the issue of asking for complaints. Asking doesn't create complaints. If dissatisfiers exist in your institution and you cannot identify them, they don't go away.

You will get more comments with more specific content if you provide a few lines soliciting them after each survey section. This helps jog patients' memories about different events and people. You'll get far fewer and less specific comments if you ask for them but once, at the end of the survey.

By getting comments as soon as possible after the patient is discharged, the experience is still fresh in the patient's mind and you're more likely to get specific, actionable evaluations. Some of the comments may be time-sensitive and reflect ongoing issues that should be resolved as soon as possible. If an outside firm manages your patient satisfaction survey, make sure you can have electronic image access to the surveys that are returned, so you can monitor comments daily. Three-month or six-month-old comments are less useful than fresh ones.

CONCLUSIONS

Don't confuse the functions of report cards and quality improvement instruments. If you must measure patient satisfaction for external report cards you still must measure it for your internal QI needs.

Patient satisfaction data are the *beginning* of the quality improvement process—not the end point. You have to begin with strength. Good data provide the tools for analyzing causes and for monitoring your QI efforts. As outside entities increasingly demand to see proof of your quality, as pressures increase for your using patient satisfaction for internal performance evaluation and compensation, you will need the best, most objective data possible.

You can collect patient satisfaction data yourself, or contract with an outside firm to do it. If you do it yourself, make sure the person managing the survey process has survey research expertise. A high school statistics course is not enough background. As we have seen, the whole process—from survey design through distribution and analysis—is a complex science. Literally hundreds of texts have been written on the subject of survey research. A lot of pitfalls can be avoided through expertise. Moreover, patient satisfaction measurement is a very special form of survey methodology. The patient is a reluctant consumer who is intimidated by the caregiver, and whose evaluations of care are strongly affected by personal belief systems.

ACTION FOR SATISFACTION

1. Keep the survey as short as possible. You can't ask everything.
2. Word the questions for patients, not for healthcare administrators.
3. Use a single response scale for ease of analysis and comparisons.
4. Ask for comments after each section of the survey.
5. Use mail-out, not phone surveys or hand-outs.
6. Keep the cover letter short, honest and to the point. No PR.
7. Send the survey to as many patients as you can. It increases the number of respondents and is good PR.
8. Mail surveys as soon as possible after patients are discharged. Next day is optimal.

REFERENCES

Dillman, D. A. 2000. *Mail and Internet Surveys: The Tailored Design Method.* New York: John Wiley.

Hall, M. F. 1995. "Patient Satisfaction or Acquiescence? Comparing Mail and Telephone Survey Results." *Journal of Healthcare Marketing* 15 (1): 54-61.

Ware, J. 1995. "Data Collection Methods." *Medical Outcomes Trust Bulletin* 3 (1): 2.

CHAPTER 5

Reporting and Interpreting the Data

You don't need fancy statistical analyses to have useful patient satisfaction data. The simplest, most basic calculations can be the basis of an effective quality improvement (QI) program.

I don't want to make analysis and reporting of satisfaction data sound too simple; it doesn't matter how simple or complex your data analyses are. If you don't use them, the data are worthless. You can do multiple regression, Chronbach Alphas, and any other fancy statistical manipulation you want. If survey results are taken seriously and responded to, the simplest mean scores and trend charts can be a powerful tool for quality maintenance and improvement.

You must be able to break your data down by nursing unit, department, medical specialty, and product line (such as Cardiac Cath Lab). For the ED you will want shift breakdowns as well. Although care does involve a system of processes that crosscut departments and units, care is managed, supervised, and effectively controlled by the separate administrative entities. Thus, data by unit and department are essential for QI efforts.

Ultimately, you will want to use a form of patient ID number to break your data down by individual physician, DRG, patient costs and charges, and so forth. In the meantime, if you know the following (and respond effectively), you can achieve high levels of patient satisfaction:

1. How are we doing overall? What does our trend look like?
2. What is scoring highest and what's scoring lowest?
   Units, medical specialties, and so forth with the highest mean scores are for benchmarking and rewarding. Those with lowest scores need fixing. (A caveat here—compare comparable elements: nursing unit to nursing unit, or physician to physician. You can't compare nursing scores with dietary scores. Dietary will always be the loser.)
3. What's changed and what hasn't since the last measure?
   A simple glance at mean scores can tell you this. In addition to looking for trends in your overall score, you need your data broken down by: individual question; nursing unit; department (housekeeping, dietary, radiology, etc.); medical specialty; and key processes (such as discharge and continuity of care arrangements; interaction with family, etc).
4. Is the change meaningful?
   You can expect some variation in your data from period to period. That's normal. If a score (for a survey item or nursing unit, for example) falls within one standard deviation of the mean, it does not differ so significantly from the mean that action is required. If a change in score clearly continues a trend upward or downward (albeit in small increments), it's probably meaningful. You don't need fancy statistics to tell you what your eyes can see over a period of time. On the other hand, a change may be unexpected and trend-bucking. Here, statistical significance tests can tell you if it is also meaningful. Can you think of any reason why the score has changed? Construction? High census? Labor dispute? Bad publicity? Reorganization of some kind? If you can find a general cause, you can then dig deeper to find root causes that will direct you to effective interventions.

5. What issues should get priority attention?

Some issues are more closely linked with overall satisfaction than others. Here you need a simple correlation coefficient. You will want to see how strongly each question is correlated with overall satisfaction. For overall satisfaction score you can either use your overall institution mean score (which is the mean for all the items on your survey) or the mean score of a single global question ("Please rate overall care you received at our hospital"). The more highly correlated the item with overall satisfaction, the more important the item. If such an item has a relatively low score, it could be having a particularly negative effect on overall patient satisfaction with care. Thus, of two items with relatively low score, focus attention on the one more highly correlated with overall satisfaction.

6. How well do we perform vis a vis peers?

You need access to comparative data to measure this. In addition to broad national information, you will need to compare your scores with those of various types of peers (identified by bed size, acuity, region, state, etc.). Comparative scores tell you how patients experience and evaluate other providers. If you are lower than they, it's a cue for action on your part. Almost all hospital administrators assume that their institution is high in patient satisfaction. Comparative data can confirm—or contradict—this assumption.

CALCULATING AND REPORTING SCORES

Your survey will probably have a 5-item answer scale, with 1 being the lowest evaluation and 5 the highest. When all the surveys are in, how should you calculate and report the scores?

You can report scores by the percentage of responses under each category. For example:

very poor	poor	fair	good	very good
2%	4%	7%	26%	61%

The disadvantage to this kind of reporting is that it makes comparisons over time difficult. For example:

This period					Last period				
very poor	poor	fair	good	very good	very poor	poor	fair	good	very good
0%	1%	7%	50%	42%	1%	2%	5%	42%	50%

Which period shows better performance? The answer is difficult, because the meaning of the different combinations is open to interpretation. When you are comparing five different numbers over two periods you are really juggling ten numbers. Is it better to have more high numbers or fewer low numbers? Comparisons can be confusing and ambiguous.

Another way of reporting scores is to combine the percentage of responses for the two top categories and simply call this the number of "satisfied" patients. Offhand, this sounds logical, but it really doesn't work. In the example above, by combining the two top response categories you would conclude that in both this period and last period, 92 percent of patients were "satisfied." Thus, no change. But is this so? Note that during this period, 8 percent fewer patients rated you in the top category. By combining the two top categories, you would never see this. Moreover, by reporting only the two top categories, you would not see the numbers of truly dissatisfied patients (Drain 2001, 44). The intensity of dissatisfaction of patients who rate you in the lowest categories (1s and 2s) has been found to be greater than the intensity of satisfaction felt by patients who give you 4s and 5s (Mittal and Baldasare 1996). Patients want to take exceptionally good experiences for granted; they never want to experience poor care. When they receive poor care, they're more surprised and affected than when they get great care.

This is not to say that "top-box analysis" has no place in your repertoire. Marketing wisdom indicates that only customers who give you the top rating are likely to remain loyal. Thus, the percent of 5s among your respondents represents that portion of your market share you can count on keeping over the long haul. All others are at risk for defection. Your goal should be to increase the proportion of 5s while reducing the numbers of 1s and 2s.

Top-box and bottom-box analyses are definitely helpful; however, the most useful scoring for ongoing analysis and improvement activities are mean scores that include all five response categories. This reflects the full range of patient experiences.

In analyzing your data, convert your 1-to-5 scale to a 0-to-100 scale, calculate a single mean score using all five response categories, and report this single mean. This process has many advantages. First, it condenses everything into a single number that is influenced by both high and low evaluations. Second, a single number is easy to compare across departments, across time or across hospitals. Third, most people are used to being graded on a 1 to 100 scale, so the reports will make more sense to your staff. Fourth, by stretching the scale out (4 to 5 becomes 75 to 100), the score becomes more sensitive. Reporting scores to the tenth of a point only allows 10 numbers between 4.0 and 5.0, but 250 numbers stand between 75.0 and 100.0. To calculate mean scores on a 0-to-100 basis, you can convert your scale as follows:

	very poor	poor	fair	good	very good
Scale on survey	1	2	3	4	5
Conversion	0	25	50	75	100

SCORE VARIANCE

Obviously, you will be very concerned with upward or downward change. How much change is significant? You probably already know about t-tests, standard errors, standard deviations, and so forth, and can calculate statistical significance. Of more conceptual importance is the need to recognize that patient satisfaction scores typically fall within a very narrow range. Moreover, this range is at the high end of the scale. Do not expect a huge spread in scores between departments, nursing units, physicians, or any other units of analysis. The reason is twofold. First, care these days really is good. Patients have great trust in healthcare providers and generally do believe that care is first rate. Second, as I've indicated before, patients are intimidated by healthcare and are generally reluctant to bite the hand that heals them.

Thus, contrary to what many people think, those who answer surveys are *not* the disgruntled complainers. Typically, 85 to 90 percent of respondents rate their care in the top two response categories. As a result, scores for most aspects of care (excepting food) tend to be in a fairly narrow high range. Your highest and lowest scores (for individual survey items, nursing units, etc.) may be no more than 10 or 15 points apart. Nursing units, for example, might typically range from a low of 78 to a high of 93. On a 100-point scale, that's not much variance. This means that small differences in score can reflect some real differences in performance. A 2-point difference between nursing units or time periods can reflect a 15 or 20 percent variance. This could be of importance when it comes to realistic goal setting.

INTERPRETING THE DATA

A brief tour through some typical satisfaction report data will illustrate their utility. These real data from real hospital reports were generated from 2000 through the first quarter of 2001.

You'll probably want to start off by asking, "How are we doing, overall?"

Figure 5.1 shows the present overall score and eight quarter trend. The overall mean satisfaction score for this period is 82.1 (on a 0-to-

Figure 5.1 Overall Mean Trend Analysis for Central General Hospital

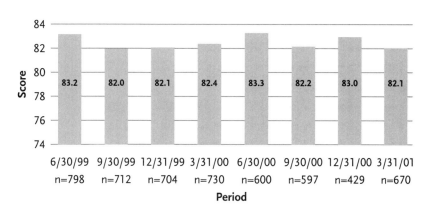

	6/30/99	9/30/99	12/31/99	3/31/00	6/30/00	9/30/00	12/31/00	3/31/01
Score	83.2	82.0	82.1	82.4	83.3	82.2	83.0	82.1
	n=798	n=712	n=704	n=730	n=600	n=597	n=429	n=670

Period

100 scale) for Central General Hospital (CGH, a fictitious hospital). The score is down almost a full point from the previous quarter. Given my earlier warning that these scores tend to fall within a narrow range of only 15 to 20 points, a drop of one point from last period represents at least a 5 percent decline. What has been going on?

Looking at eight quarters of data, it's clear that CGH is going nowhere in terms of patient satisfaction. The trend is virtually flat. Of course, if CGH's scores were the top in the country, maintaining this flat trajectory at the top of the heap would be commendable. But, as we'll see below, this is not the case (another reason why comparative data are essential).

Figure 5.2 answers the question, "What's scoring highest and what's scoring lowest?" This simple chart lists the survey item scores from highest to lowest. To save space, we have only included the eight highest and eight lowest scoring questions. As at most hospitals, physicians and nurses tend to score high at Central General. Typically, too, food and room issues fall at the bottom. Note that the lowest scoring issue is "speed of admission."

In themselves, the scores of individual survey items are not actionable. They are useful only when compared with past performance,

Figure 5.2 Central General Hospital Scores Ranked (1/1/01–3/31/01)

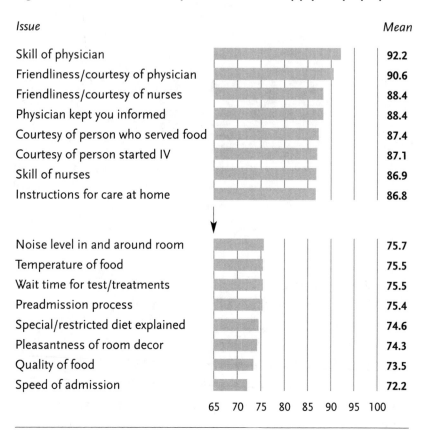

Issue	Mean
Skill of physician	92.2
Friendliness/courtesy of physician	90.6
Friendliness/courtesy of nurses	88.4
Physician kept you informed	88.4
Courtesy of person who served food	87.4
Courtesy of person started IV	87.1
Skill of nurses	86.9
Instructions for care at home	86.8
Noise level in and around room	75.7
Temperature of food	75.5
Wait time for test/treatments	75.5
Preadmission process	75.4
Special/restricted diet explained	74.6
Pleasantness of room decor	74.3
Quality of food	73.5
Speed of admission	72.2

65 70 75 80 85 90 95 100

or with external competitors, or with comparable issues on your survey. Without comparative data, you cannot really judge whether 72.2 for "speed of admission" is high or low. However, if this score represents a significant decline from last period, it becomes more meaningful. Similarly, if 72.2 is ten points beneath the national average, you've got a real problem.

Within any section of the survey there should be consistency. For example, nursing activities rated by patients include demeanor, information, skill, empathy, promptness, and response to being called. All of these constitute key elements in nursing performance. All

Figure 5.3 Central General Hospital's Greatest Increase in Scores by Issue (1/1/01–3/31/01)

Issue	Mean Last Period n=429	Change	Mean This Period n=670
Informing family about condition/treatment	82.8	+1.7	84.5
Courtesy of person who started IV	85.5	+1.4	86.9
Patient included in decisions about treatment	81.9	+1.3	83.2
Skill of person who started IV	80.4	+1.2	81.6
Physician kept you informed	86.3	+1.1	87.4

Figure 5.4 Central General Hospital's Greatest Decrease in Scores by Issue (1/1/01–3/31/01)

Issue	Mean Last Period n=429	Change	Mean This Period n=670
Speed of admission	76.1	−3.9	72.2
Noise level in and around room	78.9	−3.2	75.7
Room temperature	79.2	−2.7	76.5
Pleasantness of room decor	76.0	−1.7	74.3
Patient felt ready for discharge	84.4	−1.6	82.8

should be performed at or near the same level of quality. If "nurse kept you informed" is five or six points lower than most other nurse items, this is anomalous and should be investigated.

Figure 5.3 indicates items increasing the most. What has gone up the most from last quarter? Personnel responsible for these five issues deserve kudos this quarter. These results should be posted.

Figure 5.4 demonstrates the items declining the most. This list is headed by speed of admission, which is down by a whopping 3.9 points from last quarter. The decline is significant at the .05 level. What has happened? An increased census? A procedural change?

Figure 5.5 Central General Hospital Nursing Units Ranked (All Issues)

Unit	Mean 10/1/00–12/31/00	Mean 1/1/01–3/31/01	Change
4S	86.0	86.7	+0.7
4W	82.6	83.9	+1.3
3E	83.8	82.5	−1.3
3S	79.9	82.2	+2.3
4N	81.7	80.2	−1.5
4E	81.0	79.3	−1.7
3W	82.9	78.9	−4.0

Construction? Personnel issues (moral problems, high staff turnover, etc.)?

Also significantly lower are three accommodation-related issues—noise, room temperature, and pleasantness of room decor. Check these scores by nursing unit to see if you can pinpoint the cause. Are these low scores hospital-wide, or limited to a specific nursing unit or area? If it is not construction, get nursing and maintenance together to brainstorm.

The decline in "extent to which you felt ready to be discharged from the hospital" is likely a result of information failure, not physical condition of the patient per se. Another item in the discharge section of the survey, "adequacy of instructions for caring for yourself at home" (not shown here), declined by half a point. However, this small drop probably does not fully account for the larger "ready for the discharge" decline. Patients were likely not given adequate information upon admission about expected length of stay, or explanations about their condition and prognosis at the time of discharge, and felt less at ease about leaving the hospital's protective environment.

Figure 5.5 compares and ranks nursing units. Pretty much everything happens to patients via their nursing units. Even admitting is related to the medical specialty of the unit, bed availability on the

Figure 5.6 Mean Trend Analysis for Nursing Unit 3W

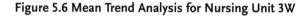

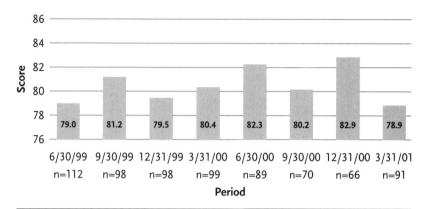

unit, signage, and so forth. Radiological exams may occur elsewhere in the hospital, but the experience is also linked to the unit through medical specialty, transport, and so forth. Food scores may vary from unit to unit depending on such things as location, and nurse protocols for tray distribution, among others.

In the figure, the units are ranked from highest to lowest overall mean score, with all items on the survey contributing to the mean. We note that 3w is not only the lowest scoring unit, but is also down a whopping 4 points from last period. What's going on? Before looking at specific issues that may be behind 3w's low scores, look at the trend.

Figure 5.6 is a trend analysis of nursing unit 3w. The precipitous decline on 3w of 4 points is *not* part of an ongoing trend. Indeed, by looking back eight quarters we see (with some peaks and valleys) a general trend upwards. This suggests that the recent dip is situational rather than typical and should be responded to with this in mind. Something very unusual must have happened to trigger such a sharp drop in one quarter. No one survey issue or even section of the survey (for example, nursing or dietary) can account for the large drop in 3w's score this period. Forty-eight items contribute toward each nursing unit's overall score. This suggests that something major happening on 3w is affecting a wide range of patient experiences on that unit.

We can get some insight by looking at specific sections of the survey by nursing unit. We'll look at two sections here, nursing and accommodations.

Figure 5.7 lists the scores for individual issues that make up the nursing section of the survey. The lowest score for each issue is in bold italic type. Why is 3w's score for nurse response to the call button so low? Both 3w and 4N (as well as 4E) have unusually low scores for nurse attention to patients' personal or special needs and nurse attitudes toward special requests, *plus* keeping patients informed. These are key interactional issues. Not surprisingly, patients also judge their general skills to be lower. What characteristics (staffing, census, physical plant, etc.) do these nursing units share? 4N is clearly not doing as well as other units on the core nursing issues. What's happening? 4N can use some attention.

Let's see whether we can focus in on the low room/accommodation scores. In Figure 5.8, the room items are broken down by nursing unit. Patients clearly do not like unit 3w, but a number of others are also low scoring. Check 3w's room scores for the last period. Is there some construction going on? Is it a particularly old unit? Why are 3w and 4N so low for room decor? Why, for that matter, is 4w so *high* for room decor? Is it recently remodeled? Are there more windows, or is the view better? Here, high scoring units could offer clues to "best practices" for others. Why would patients on 3w complain about cleanliness so much? (They also don't think much of cleaning staff courtesy.)

Not every item is of equal importance to patient satisfaction; you need to know what to focus on. As indicated above, score itself does not give you all the information. You need to know how each item is related to overall satisfaction. This allows you to "weight" each survey item. In Figure 5.9, correlation coefficients for the relationship between each survey item and overall patient satisfaction with care are calculated. Here, the mean for each item is correlated with the overall mean of the survey. The higher the correlation, the more

Figure 5.7 Nursing Issues by Unit (1/1/01–3/31/01)

	3S	3E	3W	4S	4E	4W	4N
Friendliness/courtesy of nurses	92.3	90.0	84.8	92.7	85.8	87.7	**84.4**
Promptness of response to call	83.2	85.5	**74.4**	87.2	80.0	84.8	79.9
Nurses' attitude toward requests	90.1	88.0	81.6	89.7	83.3	86.1	**81.1**
Attention special/personal needs	87.3	86.0	**79.8**	88.9	80.7	85.8	80.1
Nurses kept you informed	85.4	84.8	78.8	87.2	80.8	84.2	**76.5**
Skill of the nurses	90.9	88.8	83.6	90.0	84.5	87.3	**82.1**

(Lowest score for each issue in bold italic type)

Figure 5.8 Room/Accommodations by Nursing Unit (1/1/01–3/31/01)

	3S	3E	3W	4S	4E	4W	4N
Mean for Room Issues	*79.0*	*77.8*	*75.4*	*81.6*	*78.0*	*82.1*	*76.6*
Pleasantness of room decor	75.9	73.7	69.4	75.6	78.1	83.2	**69.1**
Room cleanliness	80.1	76.8	**72.5**	81.0	77.7	81.2	75.5
Courtesy of person cleaning room	85.9	84.1	**81.9**	87.8	84.2	88.2	82.2
Room temperature	73.2	77.1	77.2	77.3	**73.0**	77.9	77.8
Noise level in and around room	78.3	74.7	**72.5**	80.0	74.6	76.2	73.8
TV call button, etc., worked	81.5	82.5	**80.7**	88.2	81.6	85.8	82.9

(Lowest score for each issue in bold italic type)

likely that the score for that item and the overall mean score go up or down together. More highly correlated issues can have a greater impact—positive or negative—on overall satisfaction. Figure 5.9 presents only the eight items (out of a total of 48) most correlated and the eight items least correlated with overall patient satisfaction at CGH.

All items on the survey are (and should be) correlated significantly with the overall satisfaction score. Even the item least correlated with overall satisfaction—room temperature—has a coefficient

Figure 5.9 Survey Items Ranked by Correlation with Overall Satisfaction

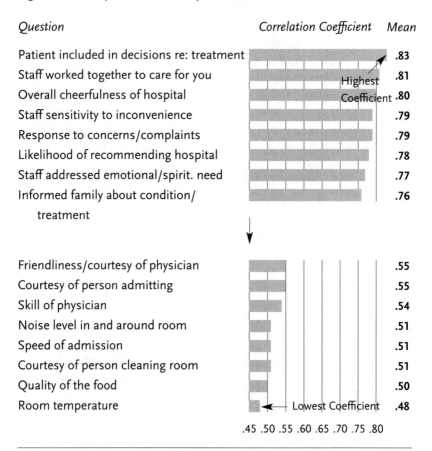

Question	Correlation Coefficient	Mean
Patient included in decisions re: treatment		.83
Staff worked together to care for you		.81
Overall cheerfulness of hospital		.80
Staff sensitivity to inconvenience		.79
Response to concerns/complaints		.79
Likelihood of recommending hospital		.78
Staff addressed emotional/spirit. need		.77
Informed family about condition/ treatment		.76
Friendliness/courtesy of physician		.55
Courtesy of person admitting		.55
Skill of physician		.54
Noise level in and around room		.51
Speed of admission		.51
Courtesy of person cleaning room		.51
Quality of the food		.50
Room temperature		.48

.45 .50 .55 .60 .65 .70 .75 .80

of .48, which is sizable. Room temperature does have an effect on the patient's overall evaluation of care. This effect, however, is far less than that of other aspects of care.

The issue of greatest potential importance to CGH patients—most highly correlated with overall satisfaction—is the issue of patients being included in the planning of their care. Patients respond positively to such empowerment. Patients also feel that coordination of care is very important. With so many staff members coming, going, and performing a myriad of tasks, patients want to know that each is aware of what the others have done or learned.

If the items most highly correlated with satisfaction are also high scoring, they can have a major positive impact on overall satisfaction. If they are low scoring, they can have a major negative impact on patients' evaluation of care.

On the other hand, items *least* correlated with overall satisfaction have less theoretical effect on it. We have already noted that "speed of admission" is the lowest scoring item on CGH's survey and also the item declining the most from the last period. However, the low, falling score must be balanced against the fact that speed of admission is one of the items *least* correlated with overall satisfaction. Thus, it may not be a high priority for "fixing." Of far higher priority should be issues that score low and are *also* highly correlated with overall satisfaction.

Figure 5.10 links both correlation and score to create a "priority index." Remember that correlation coefficients are not satisfaction scores. Items highly correlated with overall patient satisfaction can be either high or low scoring. Items that are more highly correlated with overall satisfaction and are also lower scoring have potentially greater negative impact on satisfaction and should get higher priority for allocation of attention and resources.

This table is very useful and simply created. Rank questions by score, giving highest weight to items with *lowest scores*. Then rank questions by correlation coefficient, giving highest weight to items most *highly correlated* with overall satisfaction. Finally, add the two weights to get your priority index. Higher priority index numbers represent issues with more potential negative impact on your patients' overall evaluation of care. Attention to these issues should give you more "bang for your buck."

Forty-eight questions compose the CGH survey. The issue with the lowest score is assigned a "weight" of 48; the issue with second lowest score a 47, and so forth. The issue with the highest mean score is assigned the lowest weight of 1. For the correlation coefficients, the issue with highest correlation coefficient is assigned a

Figure 5.10 Priority Index for Central General Hospital (1/01/01–3/31/01)

Rank	Quarters in Top Ten	Question	Mean Score (Weight)	Correlation Coefficient (Weight)	Priority Index (Combined Weights)
1	6	Response to concerns/complaints	81.5 (35)	.79 (43)	35 / 43 = 78
2	3	Staff addressed emotional/spirit. need	81.1 (37)	.77 (40)	37 / 40 = 77
3	1	Staff sensitivity to inconvenience	82.3 (31)	.79 (44)	31 / 44 = 75
4	2	Patient included in treatment decisions	83.2 (25)	.83 (48)	25 / 48 = 73
5	4	Overall cheerfulness of hospital	83.4 (24)	.80 (45)	24 / 45 = 69
6	4	Nurses kept you informed	82.8 (28)	.76 (39)	28 / 39 = 67
7	1	Temperature of the food	75.5 (42)	.63 (28)	42 / 28 = 66
8	1	Wait time for test/treatments	75.5 (43)	.62 (22)	43 / 22 = 65
9	3	Special/restricted diet explained	74.6 (45)	.60 (19)	45 / 19 = 64
10	5	Staff concern for privacy	83.1 (26)	.76 (37)	26 / 37 = 63
44		Courtesy of person admitting	85.4 (13)	.55 (7)	13 / 7 = 20
45		Courtesy of person cleaning room	84.7 (17)	.51 (3)	17 / 3 = 20
46		Courtesy of person who served food	87.1 (6)	.56 (10)	6 / 10 = 16
47		Friendliness/courtesy of physician	90.6 (2)	.55 (8)	2 / 8 = 10
48		Skill of physician	92.2 (1)	.54 (6)	1 / 6 = 7

weight of 48, the issue with second highest coefficient gets a 47, and so forth. For each question, the two weights for its score and correlation coefficient are added together to get its priority rank. *Score* and *correlation* with satisfaction are distinct, unrelated factors. Therefore, the item with highest priority may not be the item with both lowest score or highest correlation. The highest priority issue reflects a combination of dissatisfaction and importance sufficient to have the most potential negative impact on the patient's overall experience of care. At the same time, by improving these issues you have the greatest potential positive impact on your patients. In this example we see the ten items that top Central General Hospital's priority index, plus the five lowest (these latter are included simply to give you an idea of what's typically of lowest priority).

Heading the priority list is the issue of service recovery—how well staff respond to patients' problems and complaints. This item has the fifth highest correlation coefficient (weight of 43 out of 48) and a sufficiently low score (weight of 35 out of 48). $35 + 43 = 78$. Therefore, it has a potentially significant negative influence on CGH patients' evaluation of care. The second item at the top of the priority index is satisfaction with chaplain services. This is rather unusual. Nationally, chaplain issues are usually of less importance and relatively high scoring. Does CGH have a particularly church oriented or religiously conservative patient constituency? Is the chaplain doing something that is particularly unsettling to patients? Are staff creating expectations about chaplain services that the hospital cannot meet? (Note: As we'll discuss in a subsequent chapter, survey numbers can only identify the existence of a problem. They cannot pinpoint the causes.)

The third issue at the top of the priority index is "staff sensitivity to the problems and inconvenience that sickness and hospitalization can cause." This issue is a direct reflection of a key element of *illness* discussed in a previous chapter—the threats to role and identity caused by sickness and hospitalization. CGH's patients apparently feel threatened and perceive that they are not getting sufficient support (empathy, sick-role accommodation, etc.) from staff.

A final piece of information from this chart: For how many periods has each issue been among the top ten in the priority index? This provides insight into QI progress since the previous data period. Notice that the lead issue ("staff response to your concerns or complaints") has been a top-ten priority for six consecutive periods. Essentially, this suggests that CGH has not done much to address the issue effectively. Maybe nothing's been done at all! Is this the case?

If you can tap into an outside source for comparative data, so much the better. While internal data are essential for monitoring performance over time, they tell you nothing about the relative quality of the care you deliver. For example, your overall nursing score may be 93 (on a 100-point scale) and you may worry that it is not higher. You may want to implement programs for further improvement. What you don't know is that your 93 might place you at or near the very top of hospital nursing scores nationally, meaning that you are already great. In this case, a program directed at improving patient satisfaction with nursing would not be a wise use of QI resources, and it might have a negative impact on nurse morale.

Figure 5.11 displays the survey section scores for CGH. If CGH had no comparative data, administration might naturally focus on dietary's score of 79.8 as the lowest of its departments. It is 6 points below nursing. In truth, CGH would be wasting its efforts and resources because dietary is in the 80th percentile in its national comparative database. That's good solid performance. Nursing, on the other hand, falls in the 22nd percentile, meaning that 78 percent of database hospitals have higher satisfaction scores for nursing than CGH. Here, comparative data indicate that CGH's real patient satisfaction problem lies with nursing, not food. Because nursing contributes far more than does food to the patient's overall evaluation of care (much higher correlation coefficients), both the potential negative impact *and* the opportunity for significant overall improvement are magnified.

The more peer institutions you can compare yourself against, the more precise and realistic can be your evaluation of your own performance. If you are a small hospital in a modest-size community,

Figure 5.11 Survey Section Scores (n=684, 1/01/01–3/31/01)

Section	Mean This Period	Peer Group Mean Score	Percentile Rank Within Peer Group
Admissions	87.3	86.4	56
Nursing	**85.7**	**88.2**	**22**
Personal Issues	85.8	88.0	37
Visitors and Family	85.3	87.2	39
Physician	85.1	86.0	43
Discharge	84.6	84.4	52
Tests and Treatments	83.1	85.0	34
Room/Accomodations	81.8	77.1	88
Dietary	**79.8**	**76.2**	**80**

your effect on patients is not the same as that of a large, urban teaching institution. On average, larger hospitals score lower than smaller. Teaching hospitals score lower than nonteaching. On average, hospitals in large cities score lower than hospitals in smaller communities. Larger hospitals in larger towns have to work harder to satisfy patients. The more peer performance information you have, the more realistic will be your understanding of how you are doing.

CONCLUSIONS

As suggested earlier, some very basic data breakdowns and statistics will give you a diamond mine of information and insight. Constant review of your satisfaction data will sensitize you to changes and trends. Remember to compare apples to apples. When using internal data to note what's scoring highest and what's scoring lowest, don't look across specialties or departments. Nursing and food are not comparable. Focus, rather, on which nursing unit is highest or lowest, or which nursing item on the survey is highest or lowest.

You *can* compare nursing and food when you take external peer data into account. Percentile rank among peers is a good indicator of relative performance among your departments. If nursing is in the 20th percentile nationally and your dietary is in the 80th percentile, dietary is performing better than nursing.

Of course you want data that are statistically valid. But another form of validity is your own recognition of the truth in the numbers. Do the scores make sense? If a score goes down and you know why, you don't need statistics to tell you that what you're seeing is real. Sometimes staff attempt to cast doubt on the validity of patient satisfaction scores—particularly when their own scores are the ones that are low!

ACTION FOR SATISFACTION

1. Look at the obvious numbers first. What are the largest increases or decreases in score from the previous period? Investigate these issues. It's usually easier to identify the reasons behind larger changes. Such a detection exercise promotes confidence in your survey, as it demonstrates that the survey is sensitive enough to pick up on changes in procedures or circumstances. Your staff need to have confidence in the survey if they are to respond seriously and effectively to the data.

2. Look for trends in your data. Sometimes small changes from one period to the next are not statistically significant. But regular movement (up or down) can reveal meaningful change.

3. Use correlation coefficients and a priority index to identify appropriate targets for improvement. Issues more highly correlated with overall satisfaction have potentially more effect on the patient's overall evaluation of care. If these issues also happen to be lower scoring, their negative impact is multiplied. Attention to these issues

will give you more bang for your buck in terms of improving your overall score.

4. Get comparative data, if you can. Internal data analyses are your guide to improving performance. But you will not know whether your performance really needs improvement. If you are one of the best hospitals in the country, your patient satisfaction strategy is essentially one of maintenance rather than improvement. Comparative data tell you whether you're in the ball park or out of it, and whether you need mere maintenance or serious repair.

REFERENCES

Drain, M. 2001. "Quality Improvement in Primary Care and the Importance of Patient Perceptions." *Journal of Ambulatory Care Management* 24 (2): 30-46.

Mittal, V., and D. Baldasare. 1996. "Eliminate the Negative." *Journal of Health Care Marketing* 16: 24-31.

CHAPTER 6

Mining the Data for Insights

GOING BEYOND SIMPLE mean scores can get you closer to identifying key problem areas that need fixing or high performers that
deserve rewards. As we've seen, you can get a lot of insight simply
by looking at question means as well as unit, department, and specialty or service means. However, the deeper you go into the data,
the more specific will be your understanding of what's going on.
This chapter provides some examples of insights you can get by
breaking the data down.

Drill deeper into the data to answer some of the following questions:

- Do different types of patients have different experiences of
  your care?
- Does age or sex make a difference? Does payer?
- Is care better in certain parts of your facility?
- Does care differ by season, month, day, or time (ED shift, for
  example)?
- Does care differ by staff member?
- Does care differ by condition or procedure?

- Is there a relationship between satisfaction and profit for specific conditions?

Ideally, a patient identifier on the survey such as a bar code or number will allow you to link to patient records. With this identifier, you will be able to run satisfaction data against a host of other information about the patient. With links to records, you can run patient satisfaction against financial data (costs, charges, usage, length of stay, etc.), physician, procedure, or condition (DRG, etc.). If you don't (or can't) put an identifier on the survey, at the very least you can add a few key demographic questions that will allow you to examine patient satisfaction by sex, age, length of stay, first vs. repeat visit, ED admit, type of insurance, and so forth.

You will need sufficient survey returns to perform an accurate analysis. For example, if you get an average of 40 returns per nursing unit, you cannot break the data from any one unit down by a half-dozen patient age categories. With five or six cases in each age category, the data would not be statistically valid. However, with 500 or 600 returns for the whole hospital, most issues (and departments) will have been experienced and evaluated by most respondents. You can easily break down individual questions or survey sections by a half-dozen age categories and get good valid data.

ANALYSIS BY LENGTH OF STAY

Simple data slicing can give you a lot of useful information. The head of Central General Hospital's food service wants to improve scores. In Figure 6.1, the food items on the survey are sliced by length of stay of respondents. By and large, the shorter the stay, the less that patients like the food service. In particular, patients in for a day or less feel they have little choice of meals (menus are usually handed out on the previous day). As day surgery grows in frequency, short stays may be increasing. Providing a varied menu for same-day or

Figure 6.1 Means for Food Service Items by Length of Stay (1/01/01–3/31/01)

	1 day	2-3 days	4-5 days	6-10 days	11+ days
Information diet	75.2	77.8	78.4	80.6	79.2
Temperature of the food	76.3	76.1	75.9	77.7	76.6
Quality of the food	73.9	74.8	75.8	79.1	77.3
Received what you ordered	72.5	78.9	80.1	81.6	79.4

one-day patients may result in a significant increase in satisfaction with CGH's food.

On the other hand, note that those in for longest stays begin to find fault with the food service. This may be inevitable if your menu is on, say, a seven-day cycle. You may want to add some special touches for those patients who overlap the next repetitive meal cycle.

ANALYSIS BY AGE AND MEDICAL SPECIALTY

Here's a great example of what you can learn from drilling down into the data.

Central General Hospital had consistently low scores for skill in starting IV (Figure 6.2). In fact, CGH's latest score of 78.8 for IV starts puts them in the 2nd percentile nationally, meaning that 98 percent of hospitals in the database did better than CGH. Patient satisfaction with IV starts was fully 10 points below the hospital's mean for all other survey items.

CGH's management was very unhappy with these data. Initially, they assumed this was a technical issue and were ready to implement a costly retraining program for all IV personnel. Before embarking on this, however, the survey administrator decided to look at their satisfaction data more deeply. Management decided to test whether the ratings were age related. Figure 6.3 demonstrates that

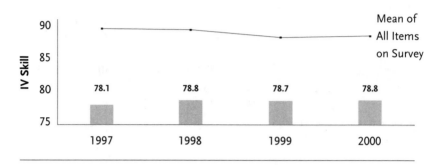

Figure 6.2 Skill of IV Starter

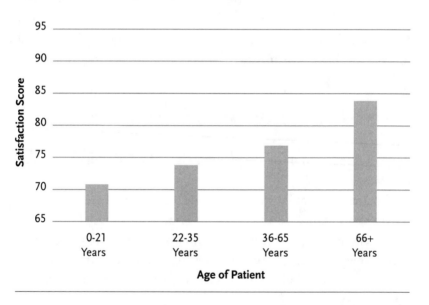

Figure 6.3 Skill of IV Starter by Patient Age

older patients' satisfaction with IV starts is well within the national average. Younger patients at CGH clearly don't like their IV starts. It makes no sense to believe that the same staff use different levels of skill with older and younger patients. Rather, older patients are likely more familiar with IVs than younger ones. Therefore, younger

Figure 6.4 Skill in Starting IV by Age Group and Specialty

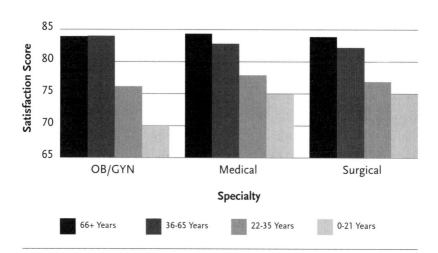

patients need more explanations about what IVs are like—where the needle goes in, how much it will hurt (or not hurt), what keeps the needle from moving around, how the drip works, and so forth.

The result of this finding was a simple in-service discussion and short brochure for nurses, stressing information that should be given to younger or first-time patients. IV start scores soared.

As long as they were looking more deeply at IV starts, CGH's staff decided to keep on searching for insights. They sliced IV start scores by medical specialty as well as age (Figure 6.4). As expected, all services showed a strong age component in patient evaluations of IV starts. Obstetrics and gynecology, however, exhibited the most dramatic age differential. Why?

It's a good bet that the older women are gynecological patients and the youngest are in to deliver babies. A staff focus group revealed that OB nurses harbored significant ambivalence about young unmarried mothers. Nurses in the unit were themselves mothers, typically with teenaged daughters. Young, unwed pregnant girls offended the nurses' moral values. Moreover, while certainly empathizing with these girls, OB nurses also felt maternal frustration at the social and economic damage that young single motherhood can do to a life. These less-than-positive feelings led to even greater reticence (and thus less information sharing) while they cared for the youngest obstetric patients. The deeper analyses of quantitative data led to a qualitative reevaluation of the OB nurses' shared value system (something very un-quantitative!). Increased sensitivity to their own value systems led nurses in OB to reshape their mode of interaction with young mothers. They might feel frustration toward some of the girls, but they could hide it better and communicate with them better. This also helped boost scores.

As I indicated earlier, satisfaction survey data are necessarily limited in specificity and usually cannot pinpoint root causes of problems. You can't ask specific questions about every possible patient experience or cause of problems. The insights to causes underlying the IV issues above came from staff, not from the survey. Identifying the age issue did not identify the root cause. Surveys only narrow the field of analysis. The data offer a *starting point* for in-house discussions and problem solving.

ANALYSIS BY PAYER

Figure 6.5 breaks down the data from CGH's emergency department by payer. Why are patients insured by insurer number 1 so much more satisfied with your ED? Why are patients insured by number 3 so dissatisfied? Your largest group of patients is insured by company number 3 (the "n" of 149 suggests this); focus serious attention on the experience of their customers (remember, *your* customers are *their* customers). Do they share a particular demographic characteristic? Age, sex, income? Do these patients tend to come from a single area of town, or from a particular local business' health plan? What clauses in their insurance might create payment problems that they blame on your ED?

Figure 6.5 Major Payers and Satisfaction in ED (1/01/01–3/31/01)

Payer	n	Satisfaction Scores
Insurer #1	61	83.3
HMO	26	81.1
Insurer #2	11	77.7
Medicare	83	76.4
Self-pay	56	76.2
Medicaid	45	75.1
Insurer #3	149	73.5

Figure 6.6 Emergency Department Physician Profiling (1/01/01–3/31/01)

Physician Code	n	Satisfaction Scores
307	22	85.9
416	40	83.9
202	62	83.3
714	47	82.9
525	12	81.8
923	260	**78.8**
491	58	78.2
350	19	**75.6**

IDENTIFYING INDIVIDUAL PHYSICIANS

Measuring ED satisfaction scores by individual physician is an example of physician profiling. With some sort of patient identifier on the survey you can identify the physician who treated the patient. Figure 6.6 demonstrates that two of your highest-volume ED physicians are among your lowest satisfaction performers. Doctor 923 is especially worrisome. He sees more patients that any other physician, and thus his low patient satisfaction performance has a big

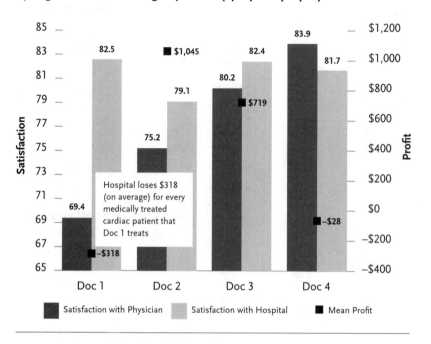

influence on overall ED score. Doctor 350 is the worst performer. Be a little careful in rushing to judgement, however, because 19 survey returns for this period may not provide a statistically significant score (when compared with other physicians). If scuttlebutt suggests that Doctor 350 is indeed bad with patients, talk the issue over with him or her and wait for the next set of scores before making an official comment or response.

USING MULTIPLE VARIABLES: PHYSICIAN, PROFIT, AND SATISFACTION

Measuring satisfaction and profit by physician allows an even more complicated and insightful analysis. Figure 6.7 looks at the medically (as opposed to surgically) treated cardiac inpatients treated by the four highest-volume attending physicians. Three variables are presented: (1) patient satisfaction with the physician, (2) patient satisfaction with the overall hospital experience, and (3) mean profit per case.

The chart is very instructive. The hospital suffers an average loss of $318 for every cardiac patient treated medically by Doc 1. Moreover, Doc 1 is clearly not satisfying his patients very well. At the same time, his patients are quite satisfied with the overall hospital experience. What's going on? Maybe Doc 1 requires a much longer length of stay than other docs (for the same types of cardiac patients) and his patients like the extended care, even though they don't like him personally. Doc 2, on the other hand, is the profit star for Central General (averaging $1,045 per patient), although her individual satisfaction scores are pretty low. Doc 3 would appear to represent the best compromise. Patients like him, and he brings the hospital a good profit and high satisfaction scores. What personal and professional characteristics does he exhibit? Perhaps he could be used as a role model for the others. Doctor 4 is a an all-around satisfaction champ, but he, too, is a money loser for the hospital. What is he doing that keeps his costs per patient high? This is a good example of how drill-down data analysis offers some specific avenues for investigation and priority setting. Let's explore the volume, profit, and satisfaction issues further.

ANALYSIS BY DIAGNOSIS-RELATED GROUP (DRG)

When looking at medical versus surgical treatment of high-volume cardiac patients, imaginative graphics can give you a lot of insight. Figure 6.8 looks at four variables: (1) patient satisfaction, (2) surgical vs. medical treatment, (3) profit per patient, and (4) volume of patients seen for each DRG. Profit per case runs up on the left, while satisfaction increases toward the right on the bottom. Volume is reflected in the size of the circle.

Figure 6.8 High-Volume DRGs by Profit and Patient Satisfaction

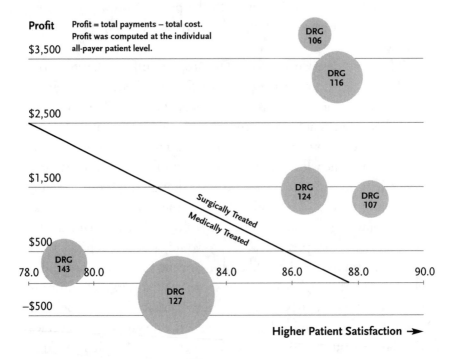

DRG 106: Coronary bypass with cardiac cath.
DRG 116: Other permanent cardiac pacemaker implant or PTCA with coronary art. st.
DRG 124: Circulatory disorders except AMI, with cardiac cath. and complex diag.
DRG 107: Coronary bypass without cardiac cath.
DRG 143: Chest pain
DRG 127: Heart failure and shock

Source: HCFA. 1998. DRG data definitions.

These represent CGH's highest volume DRGs. According to the figure, the biggest volume comes from medically treated heart failure and shock (DRG 127) but CGH is not making any money on it. Patient satisfaction, too, is quite modest. CGH has some modest profit from treating chest pain (DRG 143), but these patients are quite dissatisfied with the care.

Figure 6.9 Priority Index for DRG 127—Top Five Issues (1/01/01–3/31/01)

	Priority Index	Corr. Coef.	Item Mean
Staff response to concerns/complaints made during patient's stay	98	.91	72.0
Staff effort to include patient in decisions about treatment	96	.89	73.1
Physician's concern for patient's questions and worries	94	.86	81.0
Time physician spent with patient	90	.82	78.7
Information given to family about condition/treatment	88	.86	82.1

On the other hand, all of CGH's surgically treated patients make money for the hospital. In addition, patients are far more satisfied (by at least 4 points) with surgical treatment than with medical treatment. CGH should look more closely at big-volume DRG 127 to see what may be affecting patient satisfaction for a large number of customers.

IDENTIFYING PRIORITY IMPROVEMENT TARGETS

CGH's single biggest volume DRG was 127, and they're not doing a good job satisfying patients. To get more specific information about where to focus improvement efforts, look at data from surveys filled out by patients with DRG 127. Then create a "priority index" out of all the survey questions (see Figure 5.10). Items scoring lower, but that are more highly correlated with overall satisfaction, rank higher in priority.

Figure 6.9 is the priority index for DRG 127. The first column is the combined priority index for the item. The second and third columns show the figures that go into creating the priority rank. The second column is the correlation coefficient (correlation with over-all satisfaction) and the third is the mean score of the item. Figure 6.9 lists only the five issues at the top of the priority index of CGH. By focusing on these five issues, the satisfaction of patients within DRG 127 will likely be improved.

The list is headed by the issue of service recovery: "Staff response to concerns or complaints you had during your stay." This item potentially has the biggest negative impact on patient satisfaction with the way CGH manages DRG 127 and it suggests that patients experience problems while being treated and don't particularly like the way the problem is resolved (if at all). But what problems are we talking about? The item that is a close second for priority reflects empowerment. Would patients continue to feel that their problems went unresolved if they had more participation in their own medical management?

By focusing on the surveys of DRG 127 patients, we could look for the lowest-scoring items and assume that these issues generated problems that went unresolved. We could run correlation coefficients between the service recovery question and all other items on the survey, to see which are most highly linked with service recovery. These issues (if low scoring) likely underlie the low score for "staff response to problems or concerns." Staff brainstorming or even a focus group of patients treated for DRG 127 might help CGH arrive at a solution.

Again, I must stress that surveys alone cannot identify the root causes of low satisfaction scores. Once you have identified the existence of a problem, identifying the underlying cause and an effective solution are up to you.

CONCLUSIONS

The deeper you dig into satisfaction data, the more insights you can derive. Through a series of demographic questions on the survey itself, you can generate basic data on patient age, sex, payer, length of stay, and so forth. When you run these against patient satisfaction, you can get closer to identifying the root causes of problems. This saves time, money, and personnel and lets you be more effective in your improvement programs.

To analyze patient satisfaction data by physician, DRG, MDC (major diagnostic category), usage, and costs, you'll need to include an identifier on the survey so you can access data derived from specific cases. (Of course, you will analyze and report these analyses in the aggregate, not by individual patient.) By knowing what patients think of services that generate your greatest volume and profit you can protect your bottom line and market share and improve care for the maximum number of patients.

Note: *Of course your core mission is to provide care for sick people, not to make money,* but if you cannot sustain market share or keep out of the red, you will not be around to provide care, regardless of how high its quality. Thus, being able to link profit and patient satisfaction to specific conditions or procedures provides important insights for priority setting. Don't apologize for selecting QI targets based on volume. Improving the quality of care for *any* condition is justified and laudable—especially if your efforts affect a larger number of patients.

ACTION FOR SATISFACTION

1. Include a patient identifier—possibly a bar code or number—on each survey.

2. Ask a number of demographic questions on age, sex, and so forth if you can't use an identifier so you can do some quick, easy, in-depth analyses without having to go to archived records for these data. However, be careful not to stray into market research territory. Avoid questions that solicit income or other kinds of information that suggest the survey is less for quality improvement than sales improvement.

3. Examine low-scoring items by the demographic data. This helps zero in on causes of problems. Say, for example, that patients who rate you lowest for a particular issue are women between the ages of 30 and 50. This may give you a clue to directions for satisfaction improvement efforts. If you still can't figure out why these patients are dissatisfied, at the very least you have a good idea of the most effective composition of a focus group.

4. Analyze satisfaction data by clinical (DRG, etc.) and financial (profit, costs, usage, etc.) data. In addition to the insights previously mentioned, you will be able to quantitatively demonstrate the link between patient satisfaction and bottom line. This helps legitimize the place of patient satisfaction within the core organizational culture. Demonstrating these links can encourage commitment by showing that the payoff for attention to patient satisfaction is "hard," rather than merely "soft."

CHAPTER 7

From Data to Action

"You can't fatten the cow by weighing it." If you don't have an effective program for addressing and improving patient satisfaction, you won't get any benefit or joy from measuring it. You cannot blame the survey for low scores; to that end, this chapter focuses on problem solving and offers five ways to avoid common pitfalls in program implementation.

DON'T SHOOT THE MESSENGER

Here's the most common way in which Press, Ganey loses clients. Someone from the hospital calls us up and says, "Hey, how come our scores haven't gone up in the two years we've been using you guys to measure our patient satisfaction? Maybe we should contract with another firm!"

When we ask what they've been doing with the data all this time, they typically say, "We look at it and send it to department heads and managers." We ask, "What do the department heads do with it? Is there some particular protocol they must follow when they receive the quarterly data?"

"We don't tell them what to do. It's up to them." The managers apparently look at the reports and then file them. In short, this hospital definitely measures patient satisfaction—but that's all.

I recently got a call from a client telling us that they wanted to leave for another satisfaction measurement company. Their scores had been relatively flat for several years and they were becoming discouraged. A committee decided that the patient satisfaction survey was not "sensitive" enough. As an example, they discussed the question asking how well your pain was controlled. The client said that nurses believed the appropriate way to word this question is how well your pain was *managed*. "Managed" was a medically relevant term to nurses. They argued that pain could not be completely avoided for some conditions or procedures. "Managed" suggests a more realistic handling of pain. "Controlled," they noted, suggests full remission of pain, which could be unrealistic.

I decided not to go into all of the reasons why their contention made little sense. I did not say that the clinical implication of the word "manage" is not familiar to patients, while "control" is familiar to all. I did not point out that if pain were not fully relieved, patients would score that question low regardless of which word was used. On the other hand, if patients were given realistic explanations of expected pain and the limitations of analgesic methods, the scores would be higher regardless of which word was used.

In short, this hospital's administration believed that satisfaction scores would increase if the questionnaire were worded differently. The *questionnaire* was to blame for their flat scores. If the questionnaire were different, the patients would be more satisfied (maybe their pain would even go away!), and the hospital would not have to lift a finger to improve anything.

Of course, I couldn't say all this. It was a clear case of "shooting the messenger." I did not want to confront them about spending more time criticizing the survey than responding to the data.

The point of these examples is clear. *Measurement isn't management.* Satisfaction data provide a starting point only, then the real work begins. The best data in the world are worthless if not taken seriously or not used. Mary Malone (executive director of Press, Ganey's Consulting Services) wryly notes that

> Over the past ten years I've gotten various calls from hospitals demanding an explanation for their satisfaction scores. They say, "Our scores are down and we don't know why!" At the same time, in all those years not one ever called me to say, "Our scores are *up* and we don't know why!" Frankly, they're not calling us because they know *why* their scores are up. Up or down, they don't know why because they never investigate. When they're doing well they take it for granted. They don't attempt to find out what they're doing right so they can duplicate it in problem areas or if their scores start to take a dip. When they're doing poorly, they call us rather than turn inward to identify and address problems.

GO BEYOND THE NUMBERS FOR INSIGHT

Survey data are limited by the number and specificity of questions that are asked. Insight is also limited by the number of demographic and other pieces of data you collect from patients. Combining your survey data with other patient data may tell you that younger female patients with a particular DRG and shorter length of stay are more dissatisfied than others. But this still does not pinpoint the effective cause of dissatisfaction.

The bottom line is this: When you've finally wrung all the data dry, dug into the numbers, and mulled over the comments—the solution to the problem rests with you, not the survey.

Brainstorming When the Patient "Gets It Wrong"

To the patient, perception is reality. Let's say that patients are giving you low scores for "how well your pain was controlled." You've reviewed your procedures and come to the conclusion that nurses are indeed following state-of-the-art protocols for pain management. Is the patient simply wrong? Maybe, but that's irrelevant. Regardless of what's "really" happening, patients will still tell others that your staff don't care enough about their comfort.

With the data in, it's time to brainstorm. Discussions with staff may suggest that what's really going on is that patients are not informed sufficiently about the kind of pain that is common with their condition and the limitations of medications for that pain. Thus, their expectations are unrealistic. You cannot get this insight directly from a single pain control question on the survey. Of course you could ask several additional pain-related questions, but there's no guarantee that patients' perception of pain management will be limited to these issues. Certainly patients will not be able to judge behind-the-scenes decisions or practices that result in perceptions of insufficient pain control.

One hospital was getting frequent negative comments and low scores for daily cleaning of rooms. At the same time, housekeeping staff insisted that the rooms were adequately cleaned. They distrusted the survey data and complained about the numbers. They felt that either the patients or the data were "wrong."

The survey manager at the hospital sliced and diced the data, but the only potentially meaningful pattern that emerged was an indication that the bulk of low scores and negative comments came from several units in the hospital's older wing.

It was time to go beyond the data. A discussion group was formed with nursing and housekeeping staff from the low-scoring units, plus a few housekeeping staff from other units. Then a tour of the target units was organized. Back around the table, the group dismissed the possibility that patients were judging the rooms to be "dirty" because they were older. Although the wing was indeed older, it had been recently refurbished and had bright colors, cheerful decor, good floor coverings, windows, and so forth. The rooms didn't look or feel "old." It was also found that staff who cleaned these units also cleaned other hospital units that had high scores for cleaning. So it did not appear to be a staff competence issue.

One thing about the units did stand out, however: The rooms were organized in pairs. Two private rooms shared a common bath. In discussing the procedures that were typically used, it was discovered that housekeeping personnel entered one room, cleaned it, went into the bathroom and cleaned that, then entered the adjoining room (from the bathroom) and cleaned it, finally departing through the corridor door of the second room.

A lengthy discussion suggested that two things might be happening: (1) when staff departed the first room via the bath, the patient perceived no clear "closure" of the act of cleaning; and (2) by entering the second room via the bath, the cleaning person somewhat compromised the second patient's privacy. This brainstorming led to a simple solution. After cleaning the first room and bath, the housekeeping staff member exited that same room and was scripted to say, "There, your room's clean. Is there anything more I can do for you?" This clearly informed the patient that the room had been done (closure). By entering the second room through the corridor door, the perception of privacy-intrusion was eliminated. Housekeeping scores rose and negative comments declined.

An Exercise in Problem Solving

You have low scores for promptness of nurse response to the call button. You drill down into the survey data to see if the problem is ongoing or seasonal, gender or age related, widespread or limited to a few nursing units. After you've exhausted insights from the data, bring your own insights to the table.

Constructing a "fishbone" chart is useful in organizing a search for causes of a low-scoring issue. The design of the chart is important, as the organizing categories you choose (the major "bones") will invariably direct your thinking to causes that fit the categories.

Regardless of the specific issue to be tackled, your fishbone chart should begin with two major categories or divisions: "hospital causes" and "patient causes." Hospital causes are under the control of the institution. Patient causes refer to characteristics of patients that could affect their perception of care. Subcategories should reflect major logical elements. Hospital causes can be broken into three major subcategories: organization, environment, and personnel. Patient causes can be broken into three causal categories: condition, culture, and personality.

Hospital "organization" refers to roles, rules, rituals, job descriptions, and processes by which staff get things done. "Environment" refers to the ways in which the physical plant (rooms, layout, construction, ambiance), machinery, and objects affect what gets done. "Personnel" refers to staff personal values and characteristics resulting from race, ethnicity, social class, professional identity, past experiences, and personality.

Patient "condition" refers to both the specific medical problem (the treatment and prognosis of which could produce varying degrees of anxiety) as well as the physical condition which itself can produce discomfort and disability as well as resulting anxiety. "Culture" refers to the beliefs, practices, and expectations about health, treatment, and patienthood that the patient brings to the hospital. Ethnic group identity can play a large role here. As indicated in an earlier chapter, these beliefs and expectations can clash with standard clinical values and practices. "Personality" refers to idiosyncratic personal characteristics brought to the hospital. These characteristics can result from patient age, sex, professional or domestic identity, past experiences, and so forth.

In any instance where patients give you a low score, assume that the cause can lie either with you or the patient, or both. With the major "bones" identified, you can more easily identify specific situations or behaviors that can cause the problem.

The cause-and-effect fishbone diagram in Figure 7.1 does not identify all possible causes, nor are all the categories listed relevant

Figure 7.1 Cause-and-Effect Fishbone Diagram

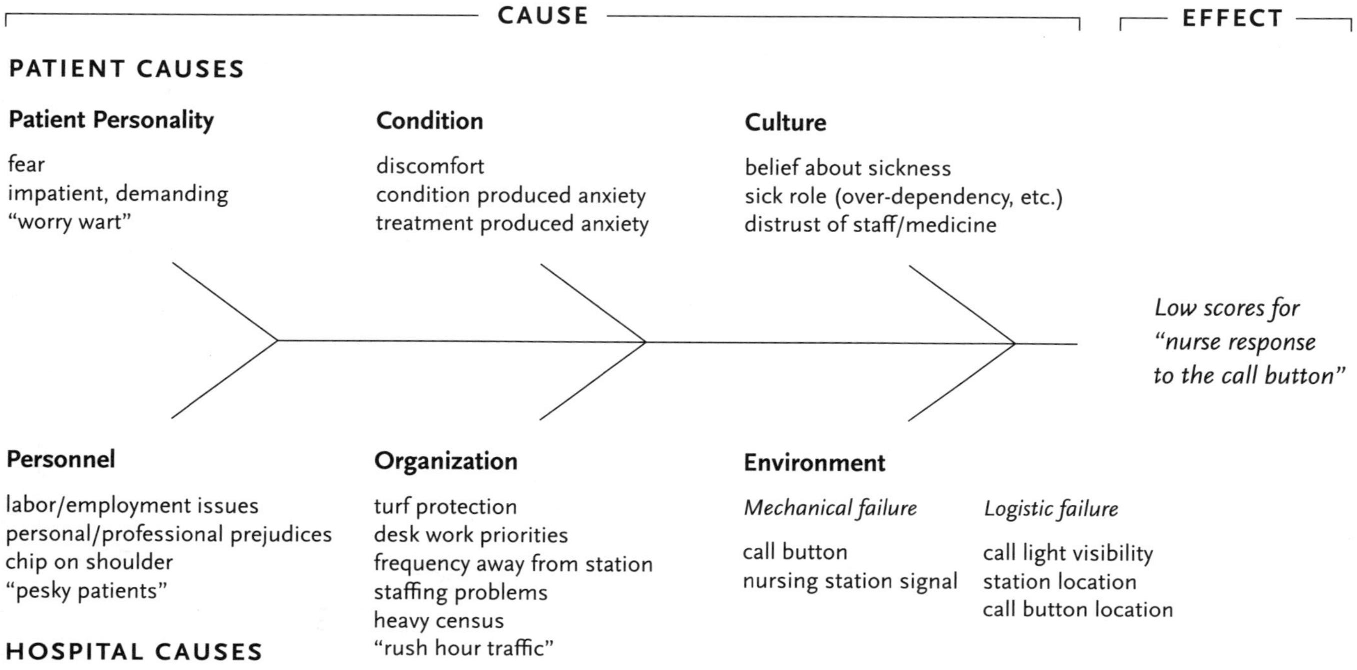

CAUSE — — EFFECT

PATIENT CAUSES

Patient Personality

fear
impatient, demanding
"worry wart"

Condition

discomfort
condition produced anxiety
treatment produced anxiety

Culture

belief about sickness
sick role (over-dependency, etc.)
distrust of staff/medicine

*Low scores for
"nurse response
to the call button"*

Personnel

labor/employment issues
personal/professional prejudices
chip on shoulder
"pesky patients"

Organization

turf protection
desk work priorities
frequency away from station
staffing problems
heavy census
"rush hour traffic"

Environment

Mechanical failure
call button
nursing station signal

Logistic failure
call light visibility
station location
call button location

HOSPITAL CAUSES

to your institution. You will be able to add a number of other categories.

Patient causes have an effect on patient perceptions that nurses are not responding quickly enough to the call button. These perceptions may or may not be realistic. "Hospital causes" reflect genuine delays in response that are ostensibly within the control of the institution. Often, delays may not be substantial, but are viewed as such by anxious patients. Thus, delays are both real and perceptual at the same time. The solution would involve both interaction with the patient plus organizational, procedural, or mechanical change by the hospital.

For each possible cause, develop several possible solutions. For example, hospital environmental causes may involve a broken call button. Check daily to see if they are all in working order. Does the call signal outside the door or at the nursing station sometimes fail? Can nurses see or hear the signal if away from the station? Is the call button easily found by the patient? Is it part of the television control pad (thus being one button among many—patients are often confused by this)? Perhaps nurses should "test" patients' knowledge an hour or two after admission by asking them to identify and press the call button. They may have forgotten or become confused during the initial flurry of instructions and "settling in."

Invariably, you will view some "hospital causes" as beyond your control. For example, paperwork at the nursing station is continual and mandatory, consuming time that nurses could otherwise spend with patients. Unanticipated staffing shortages or an unusually high census cannot be controlled. Nurses are frequently called away from the station (for totally legitimate reasons) and may not see or hear the call signal.

Are these delay-producing situations thus beyond reach? Not if you want to modify their negative effect on patients! Nurses could carry call beepers. Protocols could be developed that allow any hospital employee in the vicinity (not just nurses) to answer a call button. Situationally high census could result in the hiring of additional agency nurses—if the hospital is willing to hit the budget for the expense. Remember that all work rules and protocols are culture— a product of decisions and rituals—and thus subject to modification.

Using Comments that Patients Write on Surveys

Comments written by patients are essentially the simplest, most direct and universally comprehensible pieces of data on the survey. Comments can be invaluable. Usually they are short and pretty general ("Nurses were great!"). Often enough, however, they are specific and go into some detail about a good or bad experience with named procedures, individuals, or types of staff.

Written comments by patients help you identify specific problems as well as processes that are working especially well. Each department and unit should receive copies of all comments, both positive and negative. Posting surveys bearing positive comments in a place where both staff and patients can see them serves to reinforce the culture. Schedule periodic sessions in which staff discuss the negative comments and attempt to identify underlying causes.

Few comments on returned surveys actually name specific staff members. If a specific staff member is named in a negative comment, it's not necessary to confront the issue unless it appears to be a pattern. If several different patients make the same complaint, the staff member's supervisor should discuss the issue with him or her.

Positive comments that identify an employee by name should always be sent to the top executive officer, who in turn should send a brief congratulatory note to the employee. (At most, a couple of these might arrive each day. Writing such notes will not compromise an executive's time.) If nurse Judy on 3w receives a copy of the survey bearing the positive comment, with a congratulatory scribble from the CEO, this is powerful reinforcement indeed—and it costs nothing.

You can use a word processing program with your survey comments to seek out keywords (procedures, physicians, nurses, units, services, etc.) that help you identify targets for reward or improvement.

SET GOALS FOR PATIENT SATISFACTION

When you have identified the possible cause underlying a problem, you will then develop a plan of action for improvement. To monitor your plan you'll need to establish goals. This is especially necessary if staff performance evaluation and/or compensation are based to some extent on patient satisfaction scores. Some issues that concern goal setting:

1. *Never set satisfaction score goals without first establishing a plan of action that should have an effect on the scores; otherwise, expect frustration and disillusionment.*

2. *Make the timetable realistic.* Make sure you establish a realistic timetable for realizing your goals. Several measurement periods may be required to implement changes and give them a chance to begin having their full impact on patients. If you note a low-scoring item in your latest quarterly data report and subsequently implement problem-solving and QI activities, you've got to give the team time to get up to speed. Do not expect to see an improvement in scores three short months later. Sometimes longer-term goals are appropriate. Short-term goals are useful only where obvious quick fixes are possible and where there is enough time for the fix to be picked up by the survey.

3. *Make the goal itself realistic.* Regardless of the method and the timetable, the goal itself must be realistic. It's easy enough to say, "we want to be the best in the country," but achieving it may be all but impossible. Whether your overall satisfaction score is based on

a single question or is derived from the scores of all the individual questions on the survey, you will have to address dozens of subsidiary issues to improve the overall score. Thus, improvement in overall score is harder to achieve. Improvements in individual survey items are easier and quicker to attain. Setting overall improvement goals of half a point to a full point is realistic. For specific, individual issues, setting improvement goals of two or three points is realistic.

It's also unrealistic to expect all aspects of the patient's hospital experience to provide 100-percent satisfaction. You will never get food scores to equal nursing scores (if you do, there is something very wrong with your nursing!). You cannot legitimately compare lab with nursing, or physicians with admitting. Patients encounter each of these with different expectations and evaluate each on a different basis. Keep departmental evaluations separate. Pit food service satisfaction scores against peer group food scores or your own past food scores, not against present nursing scores.

4. *Don't go for the big Kahuna.* Again, use external information cautiously. Don't focus on the highest score achieved nationally and adopt it as your own goal. Hospital culture, size, location, community, patient constituency, and many other factors affect patient satisfaction. For example, there is a difference of three to five points in overall satisfaction scores between the smallest and largest hospitals. The same goes for hospitals in small towns versus large urban centers. Setting extremely aggressive goals by attempting to match scores of institutions with different demographic characteristics might lead to frustration and reduced commitment on the part of your staff.

A good way to use peer achievements as a goal is to focus on improvement per se, rather than on achieving a particular score. If you have an external provider, ask them to identify the score improvements over the past year of, say, five peer hospitals (matching yours in demographic characteristics). The hospitals need not be identified. Some of them might even be relatively low scoring, but have improved significantly. Use the average improvement achieved by those five hospitals as your own goal. If they can improve "information you were given about caring for yourself at home after discharge" by 3 points, you can do it, too!

Set realistic goals that are achievable. Focus on a limited number of issues at a time. The more specific these issues are, the more chance of success. Remember that your goals may change with time. At first, goals will likely be internally guided. In a second phase, you might want to focus on issues that have an effect on your positioning among peers. In a final phase, after you've improved and your satisfaction scores are beginning to level off, focus on maintaining, rather than improving your performance; this may involve "tweaking" rather than significant intervention. Hospitals near the top in performance may have difficulty sustaining the excitement and commitment that drove earlier phases of the improvement plan. Constant reaffirmation may be needed. Bold improvement plans are far less important than motivational programs.

5. *Set interim goals.* Establish a series of smaller goals rather than aim strictly for the top. Interim goals have the advantage of being more readily achievable and give staff some continual reinforcement along the way to the top. Thunderbird Samaritan in Phoenix threw a "50's party" when they hit the 50th percentile in their peer group, a "60's party" when they hit the 60th, and, subsequently, a 70's event where the CEO donned an Elvis costume. This is strong reinforcement that keeps goals—and their achievement—continually fresh.

6. *Establish internal goals: Pick a number.* You can base goals on either internal or external referents. Internal referents are your own institution's previous satisfaction scores. Goals are set by establishing target increases for the next measurement period. You can pick an arbitrary target number or one that represents a particular percentage increase over the previous score.

Keep in mind that the range of scores is typically narrow. Within any given hospital, for example, a ten-point difference might be all that separates the highest and lowest scoring nursing units. Don't pick an unrealistically large jump as your goal. If you have a nursing score of 82, setting a goal of "10-percent increase" means a whopping (and unrealistic) 8-point jump. If your usual spread of nursing scores is, say 10 points, 8 points would actually constitute an 80-percent increase! With a ten-point spread, a more realistic "10 percent" goal would be only a single point.

6. *Pick a statistically significant increase.* Pick a number that represents a statistically significant increase over the previous score. In this case, t-tests are used to identify target numbers that represent confidence levels of .1, .05, .01, and so forth. Hitting these targets indicates that your numbers are 90, 95, or 99 percent likely to be "real" rather than a result of chance fluctuation.

If you are measuring satisfaction quarterly, your score from one quarter to the next may go up in increments too small to reflect statistical significance. At the same time, the increase over a full year may become significant.

As a general rule of thumb, the more surveys you get back, the tighter your confidence intervals, meaning a smaller increase will be statistically significant. If you are working with 200 returned surveys, an increase or decrease in score of 2 or 3 points from the previous period may not be statistically significant. With 400 or 600 returned surveys, however, a variation of but one point might indicate you had achieved your goal—or identified a problem. Remember that we're talking about the actual number of surveys returned (the "n"), not the percentage of the sampled patients who return the survey (the "return rate").

7. *Focus on reducing dissatisfiers.* You can also set goals based on something other than mean scores. For example, your patient satisfaction survey probably uses a 5-point scale (very good to very poor, excellent to poor, etc.). If you have a "very good–good–fair–poor–very poor" answer scale, monitor the number of "poors" and/or "very poors" each quarter and set a goal of reducing them by, say, five or ten percent.

8. *Quantify written comments for goal setting.* Quantify the comments that patients write on their returned surveys by simply counting the number of positive and negative comments. This can be done for the whole hospital or for individual questions, departments, or units. If the ratio of positives to negatives is, say, 4.3 to 1, set a goal of improving the ratio by 10 percent (4.7 to 1).

9. *Establish externally based goals.* Establish goals by attempting to achieve a particular ranking among your peers. For this, subscribe to an external satisfaction measurement service that can provide you with access to its national database. The satisfaction scores for most hospitals (as with any frequency distribution) cluster around a national mean. As mentioned above, this mean tends to be fairly high and the range of scores fairly narrow.

Thus, if you're one of the many hospitals clustering between, say, the 40th and 60th percentiles, a tenth of a point up or down in your mean score could move you up or down quite a few percentage points in the database (this depends, of course, on how large the database is). Toward the upper and lower ends of the national distribution, scores tend to spread out more. This means that you will need more improvement to move from the 80th to the 90th percentile than from the 40th to the 50th percentile. Obtain from your satisfaction measurement provider a printout that shows the mean score associated with each percentile position within its national database. This will allow you to set a percentile rank goal that reflects a realistic and achievable improvement in your mean score.

Externally based percentile ranks actually offer a useful and valid way of comparing very different services. Food service scores, as were noted, will always be lower than nursing scores, and the two cannot be legitimately compared. Your food scores may be 6 or 7 points lower than your nursing scores, but if your nursing scores put you in the 22nd percentile nationally (against other hospitals' nursing scores), and your food service scores are in the 80th percentile, your food service is outperforming your nurses (recall Figure 5.11).

Knowing this, set more aggressive goals for nursing and less aggressive ones for your dietary department. Dietary is already doing well.

CONCLUSIONS

If you are using sound, adequate survey methodology and have some low scores, avoid the temptation to shoot the messenger. Even if you do trust the results, you still have to do something about them. "Measurement ain't management." The survey is only a starting point. It identifies, but doesn't solve your problems.

Patient satisfaction surveys measure patients' perceptions of care. Patients can be "wrong." They may complain about something that is not actually happening, but the result is the same as if the patients were "right." If the patient perceives response to the call button as being slow, it's slow. If the room is perceived as dirty, it's dirty, and that's what the patients will tell their friends and relatives. You measure patient satisfaction to tap patient perceptions—not "objective clinical reality." If you wanted to measure what's "really" going on, you wouldn't be asking patients. Thus, to improve satisfaction with care, you must address both the care and the patient's perceptions.

When you have designed strategies to address these issues—and only then—you can set goals for patient satisfaction. Make sure the goals are realistic and achievable.

ACTION FOR SATISFACTION

1. Involve all managers and team leaders from the beginning. This ensures that the survey itself will be taken seriously. Well before your first survey is even printed, hold discussions about the questions and what they might mean to patients. A team of nurses should go over the nursing questions, and so forth. Ask your survey director (or outside contractor) to explain and defend the rationale for any

survey question about which staff may have doubts. When staff have signed off on the survey, they cannot easily complain later that it isn't appropriate.

2. Practice problem solving well before the first survey results are in. Nurses should address each nursing item on the survey, attempting to identify causes that could underlie a low score. Be methodical in these brainstorming sessions. Have staff practice creating cause-effect or fishbone diagrams for selected items on the survey. With major discussion categories preselected (i.e., "patient causes" versus "hospital causes" and their major subcategories), staff will be less likely to focus on peripheral (or less personally threatening) explanations rather than more subtle, in-depth possible causes of low scores.

3. Make survey score goals achievable. Set a series of smaller, shorter-term, easily reached goals rather than requiring a single big leap that takes a longer period of time to achieve. Short-term achievable goals reinforce commitment by offering regular rewards. Go for half a point improvement over six months rather than a full point over a year.

CHAPTER 8

Creating a Culture,
Not Just a Program

ALL SOCIAL BEHAVIOR occurs within a cultural context. Each cultural context facilitates particular behaviors and discourages others. To effect lasting change in your institution you have to change the culture. I like the motto created by Memorial Hospital Pembroke (Florida) for their patient satisfaction effort: "It's Not a Program— It's a Culture!"

There is such a thing as a "patient satisfaction culture." It consists of organizational values, beliefs, roles, and behaviors that encourage a special connection between caregivers and patients. This special connection facilitates the flow of empathy and information between patients and all caregivers in the organization. Like any culture, its members must believe in it for it to work. "Believe in" means that the culture is taken for granted and requires no special motivation or reward. Patient satisfaction becomes automatic, it is simply "the thing to do."

You cannot mandate concern for patient satisfaction if staff think it's merely fluff. You cannot demand that staff take patient satisfaction seriously if they don't feel they will be rewarded for trying. You cannot mandate it if they perceive that the task is theirs but not an equal concern of top management. You cannot have significant improvement if the CEO is not perceived by all as the biggest promoter of patient satisfaction. You cannot have significant improvement if patient satisfaction isn't tied directly to the job evaluation of every person in the organization, including the CEO. If your department heads and your CEO don't know your latest patient satisfaction scores, you are not ready for significant improvement. If patient satisfaction is not a permanent agenda item at all meetings of all groups (including the board of trustees and medical staff), the satisfaction-facilitating cultural context is not present.

You are also not ready to make a significant impact on your patients' satisfaction if you think your hospital is different from others. It isn't!

Remember that the patient, not you, experiences, perceives, and evaluates care. Whether your facility is old or new; in an upper class neighborhood or ghetto; whether yours is a large teaching hospital in a big city or a rural institution with but a single nursing unit—all patients want the same thing from you. They want relevant, intelligible explanations about what's being done. They want competent technical care. They want prompt response to the call button. They want respect, friendliness, and empathy from nurses and all other staff with whom they come in contact. They want appropriate pain control. They want promises kept. They want tasty meals and a cheerful room. They want this and a lot more from every hospital or ED or clinic in the country. Whether your patients are predominantly sicker, older, younger, richer, or less affluent than the "average" does not matter. No excuse is valid for slower response to the call button, poorer pain management, cursory explanations, or apparent lack of empathy for the personal effects of the sickness.

I am not saying that patients at all hospitals are alike. Your patients in general probably do indeed differ from patients at other hospitals with different customer demographics. The point is that it doesn't matter. Your job is to thoroughly familiarize yourself with your particular patient constituency and shape your approach to care so that their satisfaction is maximized. If you automatically adjust your medical treatment (dosages, etc.) to accommodate a patient's diagnosis, age, weight, physical condition, and so forth, why would it not be appropriate to adjust behavioral and interactive protocols to fit patient needs that might derive from their condition, age, sex, social class, education level, ethnicity, or other demographic characteristics? You must learn who your patients are and what they want from you.

You can't blame your patients for lower satisfaction scores. Blame justifies inaction.

WHAT DO WE MEAN BY "CULTURE"?

Concern for patient satisfaction operates within a cultural context that facilitates it. "Culture" is not a simple concept. Culture is a complex bag that governs meanings, values, attitudes, and behaviors for a particular group of people.

A hospital's culture thus involves far more than a mission statement or official published policies. Staff attitudes toward each other, toward patients, and toward administration are culture. When staff say "we always do X this way," or "we don't have the money to remodel the emergency department," or "Medicaid patients push the call button too much," or "administration doesn't give a damn about the stress we're under," or "only nurses should pass food trays because nurses know what patients should or shouldn't be eating," they are talking about culture. Formal (idealized) job descriptions are culture. At the same time, the way in which jobs are *really* perceived and carried out is culture. The prejudices and attitudes (professional, racial, economic, ethnic, political, religious) brought to the hospital by staff are culture. The ways in which these prejudices and attitudes are tolerated, facilitated or minimized in the hospital setting are culture.

Here's an example of culture at work.

Jake, one of our account executives, reported that he recently visited two hospitals located in the same town. It was raining heavily when he got to the first hospital's parking lot. As he contemplated getting out of his car in the downpour, a covered golf cart pulled up alongside him. He was given a dry lift to the hospital entrance.

Once inside, he approached the reception desk. He asked if the clerk could phone a particular department head and tell her he was here for his appointment. "Sure thing," said the clerk. "And when you're through talking with her, wait here a minute and we'll get someone to take you there." The clerk looked the number up, made the call, and got someone to take Jake upstairs.

Jake's visit to the second hospital a couple of hours later was quite different. It was still pouring. This time there was no golf cart in the parking lot to give him a lift. Soaking, he ran to the canopied entrance only to find a covered golf cart sitting there, the driver lounging on the seat. "Why aren't you out there fetching people?" asked Jake. "It's raining," explained the driver.

Once inside, he approached the reception desk and asked the clerk if she'd contact a particular department head.

"Do you have their phone number?" asked the clerk.

"No," answered Jake. "Could you please look it up for me?"

The clerk balked at this, stating that she had a lot of papers to go through to find the number. Jake said never mind, and searched through his briefcase until he came across the number. He gave it to the clerk who attempted to call. No answer.

Jake said he'd just go on up. Could the clerk give him directions?

"Well, it's rather difficult," replied the clerk. "You go down that corridor there until..." The directions were complex and Jake had to ask another person along the way.

Two very different corporate cultures. Guess which hospital has higher patient satisfaction scores?

Cultures Are Institution-wide

It's no coincidence that the golf-cart valet services and the information clerk reflected a similar value system.

Cultures Are Learned

Cultures are passed from one generation or group of staff to the next through both informal and formal interaction. Each hospital has a unique culture, and this culture is learned by new employees. Employees learn the culture primarily by observing and participating in it and mimicking the other staff with whom they work. This is the real, "on the ground," everyday culture. The "official" culture is of far less importance. It is picked up largely through formal training and may have little reflection on actual daily behavior. Formal training in the absence of a satisfaction-facilitating culture will not work.

Culture Is "Integrated"

An integrated culture means that its parts are typically linked to one another. Actions (behaviors, expressed attitudes, etc.) in one part affect actions in others.

Culture Is "Patterned"

A patterned culture means that concepts and values expressed in one part of the culture are expressed in other parts as well. For example, if you provide exceptional service in the parking lot and admitting desk, you are likely giving good information to patients about their treatment. No set of behaviors within the hospital is really insulated from others. What nurses say and do on 4 West affects lab staff, transporters, admitting clerks, physicians, volunteers, administrators, and every other person who comes in contact with that unit. If you introduce cultural change in one hospital sector, it will have impact on others. At the same time, the changes introduced in one sector only could be thwarted by the existing culture in other parts of the institution. In short, changing a culture is hard to do piecemeal. Nor can you expect a successful culture change for line staff if top managers don't share the same set of expectations and values (see Sherman 1997 for an illuminating analysis of organizational changes needed to attain a new level of hospital quality).

All of this means that success is best achieved by attempting to make cultural changes simultaneously institution-wide, rather than by "testing the waters" and focusing piecemeal on individual departments or staff. If culture is not shared and valued by all, it won't work. And culture cannot be mandated. Cultures, like organisms, evolve. If you can get people *performing* the proper behavior, they will likely wind up *believing* that it's the proper thing to do. Ultimately, they will do it without thinking about it. When a behavior begins to be taken for granted, it's becoming a core part of the culture.

CULTURAL CHARACTERISTICS OF TOP PATIENT SATISFACTION ORGANIZATIONS

The following were distilled from characteristics of award-winning hospitals that partner with Press, Ganey Associates in the measurement and improvement of patient satisfaction. Some have achieved "Comeback of the Year" status from *Hospitals and Health Networks*. Others have won national awards including "Success Story" recognition from Press, Ganey for exemplary improvement of patient satisfaction.

Commitment Starts at the Top

In top organizations, the CEO lives the patient satisfaction mission, and demands this orientation from everyone else. The CEO knows the hospital's latest survey scores, including the identity of the highest and lowest ranking departments and nursing units. Patient satisfaction issues top meeting agendas and occupy a permanent place on the board of trustees' meeting agenda. The CEO is held account-able for the institution's scores. A significant part of senior man-agement performance evaluations rely on their success with patient satisfaction goals for their departments or areas. The CEO reinforces the orientation by sending a personal note to every employee com-plimented by patients in letters or surveys. The CEO provides the re-sources needed to enhance satisfaction. In a financial crunch, patient satisfaction programs are among the last to have their budgets cut.

The Organization Enthusiastically Admits that Patients Are Also Customers

No conflict exists in these organizations over this question. Everyone from car parker to chief of medicine buys in to the importance of care as customer service and customer service as care. Combining both top-level commitment and the conviction that patients are customers, Convenant in Lubbock, Texas, introduces staff to their patient satisfaction program with a clear letter from the CEO (Ap-pendix 8.1).

Service Programs and Successes Are Publicized Throughout the Institution and Beyond

If patient satisfaction activities go on behind closed doors, they will not enter the culture. Successful hospitals involve all staff through activity and publicity. Many hospitals post all satisfaction scores where everyone can see them. Positive letters and satisfaction sur-veys with accolades for staff may be pasted on walls throughout the institution for both patients and staff to see. On the one hand, such publicity provides good PR and tells patients that you really care about what they say; on the other hand, public posting of positive surveys rewards staff and further reinforces the overall importance given to patient satisfaction. Awards and recognition should be continual throughout the year (such repetitive rituals serve to reinforce the culture).

Institution-wide celebrations for improvements in overall satisfaction scores are essential. After all, everyone contributes to the patient's total experience of care. Van Wert County Hospital (Ohio) gave celebratory t-shirts to all staff when they first hit the 99th percentile in patient satisfaction nationally. The next year, when they had sustained their high-scoring position, a hospital-wide pizza party marked the occasion. Not only that, Van Wert produced several PR commercials (aired on local TV stations) proudly proclaiming their achievements in patient satisfaction.

You probably already have an in-house newsletter. Make sure that patient satisfaction stories and programs are high profile. Two hospital newsletter examples from Bristol (Connecticut) and Columbus Regional (Indiana) hospitals include patient satisfaction stories on the front page (Appendixes 8.2 and 8.3).

Patient Satisfaction Data Are Taken Seriously and Each Report Is Eagerly Awaited

Staff in every department and unit know their latest satisfaction scores and what their trends are. Satisfaction survey results are posted around the hospital and all know each others' performance.

If the survey and its scores and trends are monopolized by some central office and not shared with all staff, "ownership" of patient satisfaction cannot be institution-wide.

Each department head is responsible for an action plan to improve satisfaction and the plan is reviewed and updated at regular intervals such as 90 days. Realistic goals are set. A hospital in the 10th percentile for ED waiting time should not set a one-year 90th percentile target. If progress is not reported, a new action plan must be presented that analyzes the failure to improve and outlines clear steps for improvement. Management does not view "We're working on it" as an acceptable progress report. Staff view lower-than-expected scores as opportunities for improvement, not occasions for punishment.

Staff Are Hired and Trained for Service-Relevant Qualities as well as Task-Specific Skills

During hiring interviews, applicants are screened for personality types that reflect an openness to innovation and to appreciating the importance of the patient's views of care. Those who exhibit distrust of the legitimacy of the patient's evaluation of care are not hired. Some hospitals require new recruits to sign a pledge that focuses attention on efforts to promote quality and patient satisfaction (Appendixes 8.4 and 8.5). New hires typically sign such pledges after reviewing the behavioral standards demanded (Appendixes 8.6, 8.7, and 8.8).

During training, the fact that institutional financial survival depends upon viewing patients as customers is stressed. No beating around the bush by focusing solely on lofty mission statements. You have to stay in business, and staff should know that patient satisfaction is a key to the hospital's survival—and to their own long-term job security.

Scripting is used to standardize some mandatory aspects of staff interaction with patients (i.e., "Is there anything more I can do for you?," "Would you like me to go over that again?"). Staff are coached in presenting clear explanations for technical acts (IV starts, EKGs, respiratory therapy, etc.), as opposed to assuming that patients know what's going on. If specific technical errors are prevented through mandating protocols for treatment, so too specific interpersonal /communication errors (as indicated by low satisfaction scores) can be prevented through scripting behavior and interactions.

Scripting can be useful in every department or service. Centra-State Medical Center (Freehold, New Jersey) noted low scores for physician-related items on the emergency patient survey. The low-scoring issues were essentially interactional. For each issue, a simple script was developed to improve communication. Michael Jones, M.D., chairman of the ED, worked with staff physicians to develop a number of scripted statements. Because the importance of patient satisfaction improvement was stressed and because the effort was led by the ED chief (himself a physician), resistance was minimal. The scripts had the following characteristics:

- Easy to memorize (no need to refer to a written prompter and more likely to encourage physician compliance)
- Reflected the wording of a survey item that was an improvement target
- Reflected empathy or concern on the part of the physician

Scripted behavior or communications were created for the following five survey issues:

1. Courtesy of the physician.
   Scripts:
   a. "Hello, I'm Dr. _____, and I'm here to take care of you."
   b. Address the patient formally, not by first name.
   c. Don't ignore accompanying family.
2. Degree to which the physician took your problem seriously.
   Scripts:
   a. "I'm sorry this happened to you. We'll take good care of you."
   b. "This must have been a very (fill in appropriate word: painful, frightening, upsetting, etc.) experience for you."
   c. "I can see that you are ..."
   d. "It sounds like what you're telling me is ..."
   In addition to verbal issues, the group scripted behavior as well:
   a. Make eye contact.
   b. Nod in response, or say "uh huh" to show you're listening.
   c. If at all possible, sit. Don't stand next to the patient.

3. Physician's concern for your comfort while treating you.
   Scripts:
   a. "I see you're in pain. Let me ... (fill in what you plan to do)"
   b. "We want to make you as comfortable as possible."
4. Physician's concern to explain your tests and treatments.
   Script: "If there's anything you don't understand, please stop me."
5. Advice you were given about caring for yourself at home.
   Scripts:
   a. "Here's what you can expect ..."
   b. "Here's what you need to do when you leave here ... (clear, written discharge instructions)"

CentraState's ED scores rose significantly and other specialty areas within the hospital began to develop simple scripts for staff to use in common situations (Gutter and Marinaro 2000).

Any patient stay in the hospital involves multiple contacts and interactions with staff. The scripting described above is very useful and easy; however, it represents but a small fraction of the verbal and nonverbal communication between patient and staff. Staff attitudes, prejudices, and values, and their effect on staff interaction with patients are far more difficult to deal with. It's one thing to say "don't be defensive," it's another to actually avoid defensiveness if you feel the patient is unworthy or unqualified to criticize you. In the highly rated patient satisfaction institution, workshops are conducted on the effect of staff interaction (both content and personal style) upon patients and their families. Self-reflexive sessions are led by behavioral specialists, focusing on the impact of staff personal and professional values upon their interaction with patients. Simplified discussions on the illness/disease dichotomy are scheduled to make staff aware of the complex beliefs, expectations, and experiences brought by patients to the hospital setting. (Remember, simply saying "be sensitive to patient beliefs and backgrounds" does not tell you what these differences are or how to deal with them.) Staff must realize that patients have agendas, too, and that these consist of far more than desire for smiles, warm blankets, and a generic word of comfort (however nicely scripted).

Staff training must also involve sensitization to the elements of the hospital culture that can thwart efforts at maximizing care. The systemic nature of processes, problems, and solutions (i.e. cross-cutting departmental interconnections) are stressed. Discussions about turf and job boundaries are necessary, focusing on the disadvantage of turf protection for patients and for the hospital's mission of quality care.

All of these training elements focus on the legitimacy of the patient's perspective and its effect on care, outcome, and subsequent evaluation of the hospital experience. You also need to educate staff to the importance, legitimacy, and utilization of your patient satisfaction survey.

Training sessions for line staff on the patient satisfaction survey are best done by department or specialty. Copies of the survey are distributed, along with an explanation of methodology. Sample excerpts of the data reports are provided so staff can familiarize themselves with the numbers and how to interpret them. Staff brainstorm about possible causes and solutions for low-scoring survey items. This prepares them for the task ahead and helps demystify the process of responding to the survey data.

There is no single training model that all institutions should use. Cunningham and Malone (1999) note that at Thunderbird Samaritan (Glendale, Arizona), all employees must participate in eight hours of experiential training, focusing on compassion, integrity, and excellence. Similarly, Columbus Regional (Indiana) requires that employees take ten hours of classes dealing with the organization's standards of service. Focusing on leaders as well as general employees, Baptist (Pensacola, Florida) requires all middle and upper management to spend two days (off site) every three months, receiving training on hiring, supervision, communication, and other satisfaction-focused topics (Cunningham and Malone 1999).

When Memorial Hospital Pembroke (Florida) undertook it's "wow" Customer Service Program, it designed six educational classes that all staff members had to attend. The classes and the topics they covered were:

1. *First Impressions*
   - A video of "Do's and Don'ts"
   - "You only have one chance to make a first impression"
   - Disney's approach to impressing the customer
   - Why first impressions are lasting
   - Dressing for success
2. *Achieving Excellence*
   - Successful customer service organizations—What makes them that way?
   - What makes customer service in healthcare different
   - The benefits of customer service
   - How to get from where we are to where we want to be—and stay there
   - Begin with the end in mind
3. *Customer Service Principles*
   - Basic rules of customer service
   - Reasons why patients recommend hospitals
   - Five key concepts of customer service
   - The importance of word of mouth
4. *Teamwork*
   - Building a strong sense of teamwork
   - Working as part of a customer service team
   - Defining the essential skills needed to provide wow service
   - How to maintain a positive team in the workforce
   - Interdepartmental cooperation
5. *Effective Communications*
   - Verbal and nonverbal communication
   - Telephone etiquette

- Active listening skills
- Demonstrate to customers that what they have to say is important to you
  - Focus on the customer's needs
  - Avoid interrupting when the customer speaks
  - Verify and clarify what the customer is saying
  - Maintain eye contact
  - Ask questions in an organized sequence
6. *Resolving Customer Problems*
  - Identify reasons for customer problems
  - Why healthcare is a problem-prone business
    - Problems are the nature of our business (Patients and families come to us in an already high state of stress, the family's expectation of care is higher than the patient's, and we deal in highly complicated, confusing systems)
    - Expectations of care continue to grow
    - Increased public attention to healthcare (puts us in spotlight)
  - The common problems and how to resolve them
  - The best way to avoid problems
  - What customers want most and get the least

At the completion of the final class, Memorial invited employees to a "wow" luncheon. Reflecting the hospital's serious view of the program, it was actually a formal affair with tablecloths, flowers, china, and a fancy menu. The top administrator spoke and attendees were given their "wow" pins.

A final word about training: Don't waste the time and money if a major, institution-wide patient satisfaction program is not already underway. Don't train staff if the CEO is not visibly and obviously committed to the program. Seeds sown on sterile ground will not grow. One hospital we know of (not one mentioned above) spent big bucks on customer service training for employees, sending them in groups or individually for all-day training sessions. At the same time, no overall organizational program was in place to which all staff were committed and that top leadership actively promoted. When staff returned to their departments after the day of training, they returned to an unchanged cultural context and group dynamic unconcerned with working together to improve patient satisfaction. Needless to say, the hospital's satisfaction scores continued to be low.

Staff Are Empowered to Provide Exceptional Service

At a top patient satisfaction organization, staff feel "permitted" to spend a bit more time with patients when they judge it to be necessary. If a patient expresses a need, staff can fill it, if it's within their abilities. As Eisenberg (1997) notes, "the less empowered the employees, the greater the delay in satisfying the customer." Empowerment also entails a recognition that turf boundaries can be crossed for the sake of patient satisfaction. For example, a housekeeping staff member can refill a patient's ice water or make a phone call to a relative without feeling that it "isn't in my job description" or "I'm stepping on someone else's territory."

Some hospitals empower all levels of staff to provide at least token restitution (gift or certificate from the hospital gift shop, for example) where they believe patients have experienced some form of service failure. Employees at Holy Cross Hospital in Chicago are authorized to spend up to $250 per patient for service recovery. Staff tend not to go overboard in this and the total cost is typically negligible (the very act of empowering employees in this way creates a heightened sense of responsibility for and to the institution).

Service recovery (how well complaints or problems are handled) is one of the survey items most highly correlated with overall satisfaction with care. Service recovery is facilitated when all staff are empowered to participate.

Staff Reward Each Other for Their Patient Satisfaction Orientation

When staff reward each other for patient satisfaction, it reflects a real "buy-in" on the part of staff. Do what you can to encourage it. Many variations of this type of program exists, but the theme is pretty consistent. Staff member "A," observing staff member "B" do something special for a patient, awards "B" a certificate of recognition on the spot. Those who accumulate sufficient accolades from their peers receive a special reward from management (cash, gift certificate, write-up in the staff newsletter, etc.).

Many different names exist for these peer-recognition programs. Albany Medical Center has a "Giraffe Award," given by a staff member to another judged to have "stuck his or her neck out" for a patient. Another hospital has a "Caught in the Act" award.

At Columbus Regional Hospital (Indiana) employees can send a "Care-Gram" to another employee judged to be providing exceptional service to patients. Furthermore, when an employee is mentioned positively on the patient survey, he or she is given two carnations by the CEO. The honored individual then has to give one of the flowers to another employee who, "behind the scenes," has contributed to the exceptional service praised on the survey. (This is a great idea because it calls attention to the integrated, interdepartmental, systemic nature of care.)

Clara Maass (New Jersey) implemented a "Just Desserts" program in which complimentary dessert certificates (redeemable at the hospital cafeteria) are periodically handed out to *both* patients and staff for presentation to employees judged to render exemplary customer service.

Baptist Hospital in Pensacola developed a "wow" program that concentrated on looking for employees who provided outstanding customer service. Staff who were "caught" by their own or any other manager or administrator were recognized on the spot with a hot pink wow card. Employees receiving five wow cards were given a $15 gift certificate (to a local business) by their manager. Certificate winners' names (and the number of wow cards they've been awarded) are published monthly in the Baptist newsletter. When the program began, Baptist instituted few rules and no limits to the number of awards an employee could receive. Some staff, of course, were consistent wow winners because of their special commitment to core issues of patient satisfaction. Baptist did not worry about some individuals monopolizing the awards, because the behavior of these consistent winners could serve as a model for others.

Many hospitals have some form of wow or Care-Gram program (Appendixes 8.9, 8.10 and 8.11). The point is simple: When you encourage employees to recognize each other for enhancing your patients' experience of care, they will respond by doing even better. Peer recognition increases staff's commitment to the job and to their patients. When peers recognize each other's commitment to patient satisfaction, the culture is reinforced. The result is more satisfied patients as well as employees.

Staff Are Regularly Evaluated for Their Patient Satisfaction Orientation

Staff are not only rewarded for success, but are held accountable for decreases as well as increases in patient satisfaction scores. A portion of compensation may depend upon departmental or unit performance. Recognition that one's own performance can affect the compensation of one's peers is a powerful incentive. Part of job performance evaluations may include evaluations by staff in other departments or areas on the employee's ability to facilitate the tasks of others.

Staff Are Rewarded by Management for Their Commitment to Patient Satisfaction

Survey score increases are routinely praised and recognized. A minor budget item allows managers to distribute gift certificates (local fast-food restaurants will likely give you a bunch free) or other low-cost "perks" to their staff when scores go up. Returned surveys that praise specific staff members are posted publicly in that department. At JFK Medical Center in Edison, New Jersey, staff who receive five or more positive comments on patient satisfaction surveys (during any data gathering period) receive a "Superstar" pin from senior management. They are worn proudly.

Bonuses based on achieving specific patient satisfaction score goals may or may not be part of management strategy. It is not essential that you profit-share. Purely symbolic, nonmonetary rewards can themselves be powerful incentives for maintaining the culture. At St. Luke's Episcopal Hospital in Houston, low ED satisfaction scores spurred a broadly supported QI effort. In the first quarter following project inception, the ED moved from the 5th to the 26th percentile among EDs in the Press, Ganey national database. Even though this was still low-performing, St. Luke's president donned an apron and hosted an improvement-recognition party for ED staff. Within three quarters, St. Luke's emergency department had achieved 99th percentile status and were rewarded with a new stereo and automatic iced-tea maker for the staff lounge. These recognitions cost the hospital little, but had significant effect on morale and commitment.

When Bristol Hospital (Connecticut) hit the 95th percentile in the Press, Ganey national patient satisfaction database, their CEO, Tom Kennedy, threw a lawn party and cafeteria "sundae celebration." Again, the cost is minimal, but the impact great. The CEO's commitment is obvious.

CONCLUSIONS

All organizations have their special culture. Hospital cultures consist of all the roles, rules, behaviors, values, and opinions of staff and administration. Cultures are learned and transmitted via people observing and interacting with others, not through mission statements and edicts alone. The most effective patient satisfaction programs are institution-wide, reflecting commitment from the top to bottom. Otherwise, tension will be constant as committed elements run up against uncommitted departments or individuals who thwart the improvement processes. The goal is to make patient satisfaction such a part of the institutional culture that it is taken for granted. When formal programs are supplanted by everyday institution-wide behavioral demonstrations as the basic form of training, you've got your culture in place.

ACTION FOR SATISFACTION

1. Plan for an institution-wide, long-term program.
2. Make sure all staff play some role in improvement program planning and/or implementation.
3. Make patient satisfaction a mandatory meeting agenda item for *all* groups.
4. Emphasize patient satisfaction as a key criterion for employment, advancement, and reward. No staff group can be exempted.
5. Publicize patient satisfaction efforts and successes throughout the institution.
6. Establish mechanisms for staff to reward each other for exemplary service.
7. Give regular, publicized rewards for exemplary or improved performance. Keep the fire burning.

REFERENCES

Cunningham, L., and M. P. Malone. 1999. "Newsletters Aren't Enough: Best Practices in Internal Communication Lead to Impressive Patient Satisfaction Scores." *Strategies for Healthcare Excellence* 12 (9): 1-7.

Eisenberg, B. 1997. "Customer Service in Healthcare: A New Era." *Hospital and Health Services Administration* 42 (1): 17-31.

Gutter, E., and M. Marinaro. 2002. "The Most Powerful Drug [Is Words]." *Satisfaction Monitor* (Jan/Feb): 1-3.

Sherman, C. 1997. *Creating the New American Hospital.* San Francisco: Jossey-Bass.

Appendix 8.1 Covenant PRIDE Customer Satisfaction Welcome Letter

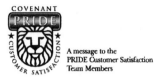

A message to the
PRIDE Customer Satisfaction
Team Members

We want to express our sincere appreciation and excitement for your participation in the Covenant PRIDE Customer Satisfaction program.

What you are about to read (and embark upon) was created by your peers – not executives sitting in an office far from the patient care front line. After talking with many of you, what we heard was that it was most important to you to be able to feel pride in the work you do because your work really matters to you.

The Covenant PRIDE program incorporates our Mission, Vision and Values into service standards, patient interaction guidelines and other elements of the PRIDE program that are outlined in this booklet. These are the "basics" for the strategy behind providing stellar care to our customers.

I strongly encourage you to have an open mind and give 100% as you embark on this program. We are indebted to you for helping us accomplish our goal of service excellence.

Chris Barnette
CHS Executive VP/Chief Operating Officer

CHS PRIDE Customer Satisfaction Vision Statement

We will be preferred and recognized for our values-based customer service by consistently achieving a patient satisfaction ranking in the top 10% of all hospitals our size.

Used with permission from Covenant Health System, Lubbock, Texas.

Appendix 8.2 Front Page of a Weekly Publication for the Employees of Bristol Hospital

Newsline

Volume XVII- No. 5 • **A Weekly Publication for the Employees of Bristol Hospital** · February 15, 1999

From the President's Desk

Friday, our "Top 5% Patient Satisfaction Bonus Day," was a memorable day for me and I hope you share that feeling. I can report that 660 fellow employees came through the old ICU and received their cash bonus award. The other 245 bonus eligible employees will receive their compensation in the form of a check to be processed this week. Many of you took the time to thank me for what was happening on Friday. But the thanks really goes to you. Everyone who works here has contributed to our success under this program. If you want to thank someone, spread it around.

A number of employees asked me for more details about exactly what level of success we achieved. Over the course of the last nine months, we have been rated in the top 5%, which means we are better than 95 out of 100 hospitals in patient satisfaction. Given that within Press Ganey we compete against approximately 500 hospital who also are striving for excellence, this makes our achievement of top 5% very special. To put it simply, we are ranked as one of the top 20 hospitals in the Press Ganey universe.

We will be using every opportunity to boast about this significant achievement and all of your efforts in the newspaper and at the Home Show. The pride that I sense as I walk through the building is very real. I sense it not just among members of the work force, but also among our patients and their families. Our community is already responding with pride at our level of achievement.

On Friday we gave staff "Top 5%" blue ribbons to wear on their badge. These ribbons and window decals are for all employees. Stop by Public Relations on Level E if you do not yet have a ribbon or window decal. For at least the next month you may

proudly wear the ribbon in celebration of our accomplishment. I have every confidence that we can keep up this great work.

If your weekend allows, please come by the Bristol Hospital displays at the Chamber's Home Show. We would love to see you there.

- Tom Kennedy

Weekly Statistics (1/31/99 - 2/6/99)	
Admissions	
Budget:	135
Actual:	153
Last Year:	157
Patient Days	
Budget:	600
Actual:	574
Last Year:	725
Average Daily Census	
Budget:	86
Actual:	82
Last Year:	104
Outpatient Services (Reg.)	
Actual:	3630
Last Year:	3928

Congratulations to Both!

Many of you may have seen the article in *The Bristol Press* about EMT William Kenney. In addition to his duties here at Bristol Hospital, Bill is a 15 year veteran of the Bristol Police Department. He was recently chosen to be the 1999 Police Officer of the Year by the Exchange Club and will be honored at a dinner to be held at Nuchie's Restaurant on February 22. Joanne Kuntz, MD, will be the keynote speaker. One of his many accomplishments is being the motivating force in bringing automated defibrillators to the Bristol Police Department.

For those of you who wish to attend the dinner, tickets are available at the Bristol Police Department , Shannon's Jewelers and the Greater

Bristol Chamber of Commerce. Congratulations to Bill on this well-deserved honor.

Shirley Breuer, MA, PT, OCS, CSCS of Rehab Dynamics/ Newington was recently certified as a clinical specialist in orthopaedic physical therapy by the American Board of Physical Therapy Specialists. Shirley is one of 1245 physical therapists certified in the United States and one of 30 certified in the state of Connecticut. To receive board certification, candidates must successfully complete an extensive examination and demonstrate specialized knowledge and advanced clinical proficiency in a special area of physical therapy practice. Congratulations to Shirley on this most significant accomplishment.

Y2K - Squash the Bug Personal Tips

The American Red Cross advises that you examine your smoke alarms now. If you have smoke alarms that are hardwired into your home's electrical system, check to see if they have battery back-ups. Every fall, replace all batteries in all smoke alarms.

Indemnity Dental Announcement

Effective February 1, 1999, a new company called The Phoenix will process your indemnity dental claims. **Your dental benefits have not changed**. Please use the forms being mailed to your home to submit claims incurred after 2-1-99 to The Phoenix. New dental ID cards will be issued by the end of February.

Additional dental claim forms are available in the Human Resources Department.

(over)

Used with permission from Bristol Hospital, Connecticut.

Appendix 8.3 Front Page of Columbus Regional Hospital's Newsletter, "In the Know"

In The Know at Columbus Regional Hospital

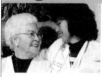

Wednesday, August 25, 1999

Know Your Customer…

Upcoming Activities

August 23 – 27 – Employee Photos Taken

August 25 – Satisfaction Fair

August 28 – Volunteer Day for Housing Partnerships

September 1 - Employee Update Session

September 4 - Hospice Concert

September 7 - Deadline to Register for Seven Habits

September 8 – Employee Picnic

Satisfaction Fair

Visit the East Gallery on Wednesday, August 25th from 8 a.m. - 5:30 p.m. for the hospital's first-ever Satisfaction Fair. Over 30 booths will be set up for departments to share how they are working to improve customer satisfaction. Prizes will be awarded and special activities are planned. Come join the fun. Watch for next Wednesday's In The Know for a review of the event.

Extraordinary Story

The following is this month's Extraordinary Story which demonstrates hospital employees who are going the extra mile to deliver outstanding customer service for a fellow coworker…

> When a sudden family crisis left Caroline McDaniel without childcare for her infant son, coworkers stepped in and volunteered to use their days off work to help out. "I was working nights and was not only struggling with child care during the night but also needed help during the day so I could rest. I could not have survived during this trying time without the help of my co-workers, and the support of my manager. I would like to recognize all 3 Tower employees for being patient with me during this difficult time. Special thanks to Brenda Murray, Anna Bunch, DeAnna Followell, Heather Welchel, Erica Jones, Beth Wright, Erin Haufe and Heather Haufe. Their commitment to me strengthened my commitment toward the hospital.

Weekly Satisfaction Score

The hospital's overall inpatient satisfaction score for the week of August 16th was a mean score of 82.8. The distribution of responses for the week was: Very Good 46%, Good 43%, Fair 10%, Poor 2%, Very Poor 0%. There has been a drop in Very Good responses down to Good, which has caused a decline in scores over the past few weeks. Continue to ask the question, "Is there anything else I can do for you?" as a way to help make a patient's experience very good.

Picnic Trivia

Q. What movie was Walt Disney's first full-length animated film?

Read Friday's In The Know for the answer and a new movie trivia question to help prepare you for the movie-theme Employee Picnic on Wednesday, September 8th. The movie trivia question on Monday was, "Which movie was the top-grossing film at the box office last week?" Answer is "The Sixth Sense." Watch In The Know for more details about picnic activities.

COLUMBUS
REGIONAL
HOSPITAL

Used with permission from Columbus Regional Hospital, Indiana.

Appendix 8.4 Pledge to Patient Satisfaction Required of All Bristol Hospital Staff

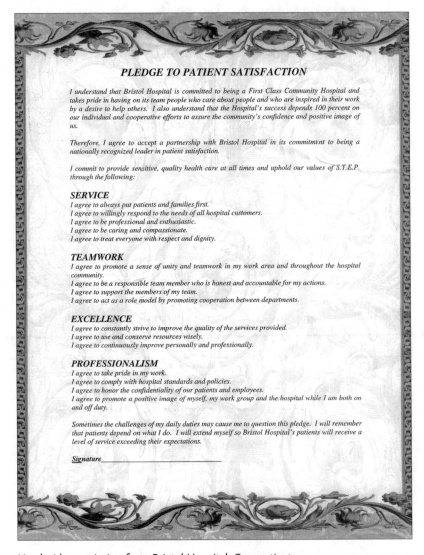

PLEDGE TO PATIENT SATISFACTION

I understand that Bristol Hospital is committed to being a First Class Community Hospital and takes pride in having on its team people who care about people and who are inspired in their work by a desire to help others. I also understand that the Hospital's success depends 100 percent on our individual and cooperative efforts to assure the community's confidence and positive image of us.

Therefore, I agree to accept a partnership with Bristol Hospital in its commitment to being a nationally recognized leader in patient satisfaction.

I commit to provide sensitive, quality health care at all times and uphold our values of S.T.E.P. through the following:

SERVICE
I agree to always put patients and families first.
I agree to willingly respond to the needs of all hospital customers.
I agree to be professional and enthusiastic.
I agree to be caring and compassionate.
I agree to treat everyone with respect and dignity.

TEAMWORK
I agree to promote a sense of unity and teamwork in my work area and throughout the hospital community.
I agree to be a responsible team member who is honest and accountable for my actions.
I agree to support the members of my team.
I agree to act as a role model by promoting cooperation between departments.

EXCELLENCE
I agree to constantly strive to improve the quality of the services provided.
I agree to use and conserve resources wisely.
I agree to continuously improve personally and professionally.

PROFESSIONALISM
I agree to take pride in my work.
I agree to comply with hospital standards and policies.
I agree to honor the confidentiality of our patients and employees.
I agree to promote a positive image of myself, my work group and the hospital while I am both on and off duty.

Sometimes the challenges of my daily duties may cause me to question this pledge. I will remember that patients depend on what I do. I will extend myself so Bristol Hospital's patients will receive a level of service exceeding their expectations.

*Signature*_____

Used with permission from Bristol Hospital, Connecticut.

Appendix 8.5 Expectations of Baptist Health System Staff

BAPTIST EXPECTATIONS

Baptist Health Systems is an organization that is committed to our heritage, superior customer service and dedication to the Christian healing ministry. This is reflected in all contacts with our patients, visitors, physicians and fellow team members. Our commitment is to provide First Class customer service and we will accept nothing less. To that end, our employees are dedicated to the following expectations:

- Every individual is uniquely created and deserves special attention and recognition.

- Every employee is totally committed to being a valued team player.

- Every employee is expected to be a First Class ambassador for Baptist Health Systems.

- Every employee is empowered and has resources to satisfy and impress our customers.

- Every employee is expected to respond promptly to opportunities which will meet the needs of our customers.

- Every employee is expected to be at work when scheduled and on time.

- Every employee is expected to follow the personal appearance guidelines and present themselves in a professional manner at all times.

- Every employee takes pride in excellence, looks for opportunities for improvement and views problems as opportunities.

- Every employee is expected to perform their job to the best of their abilities.

As a future employee of Baptist Health Systems, I understand and am willing to commit to these stated expectations.

Name: _____   Date: _____

HR-067
(11-10-99)

Used with permission from Baptist Health Systems, Pensacola, Florida.

Appendix 8.6 Covenant Health System's PRIDE Customer Service Standards

IV. PRIDE Customer Service Standards

Covenant
Health System

Service

We bring together people who recognize that every interaction is a unique opportunity to serve one another, the community, and society.

CUSTOMER/PATIENT FOCUS (Values-Based Competency)
- Anticipate and strive to understand the unique needs of those serving as well as those served.
- Respond to the needs of those served and demonstrate concern for meeting those needs.
- Tailor each interaction to the specific needs of the person and/or situation.

★ ★ ★ ★ ★ ★ ★ ★ ★

SERVICE STANDARD 9

Anticipate the wants and needs of those served.

- Be aware of and sensitive to the different cultures and religious beliefs of others.
- If delays are anticipated, communicate it to the patient. If there are delays do not place blame – NEVER SAY *"We are short-staffed."*
- Be sensitive to patient needs such as hearing impairments, language barriers and disabilities.
- Focus on the education, comfort and privacy needs of patients before, during and after treatments and procedures.
- Always provide patients with blankets during transports to ensure warmth and dignity.
- Survey the patient environment and be sure to ask if there is anything you can provide to make them more comfortable.
- Listen. When people complain, don't be defensive. Hear them out and show understanding. Do all you can to make things right.
- Put the patient and family at ease. Reach out with friendly words and gestures.
- Show concern for the well being of others.

★ ★ ★ ★ ★ ★ ★ ★ ★

CHS PRIDE Customer Satisfaction Vision Statement

We will be preferred and recognized for our values-based customer service by consistently achieving a patient satisfaction ranking in the top 10% of all hospitals our size.

Used with permission from Covenant Health System, Lubbock, Texas.

Appendix 8.7 The Beaumont Standards

The Beaumont Standards

The Beaumont Standards will be known, owned and energized by all Beaumont employees.

Service

Wait times – Make every effort to provide prompt service.
- Apologize for any delay in service.
- When a delay occurs, update patients regarding their status at least every 20 minutes.
- Once service is rendered, thank patients for waiting.
- Update family members at least hourly when patients undergo a procedure.
- When interruptions occur while providing service to patients, complete their service first before moving on.
- Ask permission before placing telephone callers on hold; thank them for their patience when you return to the telephone.

Information - Provide clear explanations and accurate information.
- Explain what service you will be providing and what to expect next.

Response - Respond promptly to those requesting service.
- If you cannot perform the requested service immediately, provide a time frame for completion.
- If a request for service cannot be completed by you, refer it to the person who can.
- Answer telephone calls within three rings.
- When answering the telephone, identify your department, yourself and ask, "How may I help you?"
- If a patient's call light goes on, anyone is responsible to respond regardless of job classification.
- Respond to call lights with, "How may I help you?"
- Inform your patients when you will be away for a break or meal and when you expect to return.

Ownership

Directions – Offer to escort others who appear lost and need assistance.
- Personally escort lost people to their destination or find someone who can.
- When giving directions with hand gestures, use two-finger or full-hand gestures.

Teamwork – Show your pride in being part of the Beaumont team.
- Be a positive ambassador of the hospital in what you say and do.
- Pick up litter and report spills.
- Return all items or equipment to their proper place.

Attitude

Image – Observe the highest standards of grooming; dress professionally as appropriate to your discipline.
- Wear your Beaumont ID badge exposed at all times, either in the breast pocket area or on a provided ID badge necklace.
- Dress according to dress code.

Courtesy – Project the image that you are eager to help and that serving others is never an interruption.
- Respond with expressions such as "certainly," "I'd be happy to" or "my pleasure."
- When transporting patients in wheelchairs, face them toward the elevator door.
- Offer to exit an elevator or wait for another elevator so patients on stretchers may be transported first.
- End service interactions with, "Is there anything else I can do for you? I have time."

Respect

Introduction - Introduce yourself by name and function.
- Acknowledge others with a verbal greeting, eye contact and appropriate gestures.
- Smile and introduce yourself by your name and function.
- Address patients and families by their name and appropriate title (e.g. Mr., Mrs.) unless invited to use a more familiar name.

Confidentiality – Hold all patient and employee information in the highest confidence.
- Access only information that is essential to your job.
- When discussing sensitive matters, seek a private location.

Dignity – Provide privacy; respect cultural and spiritual values.
- Knock or ask permission before entering.
- Close doors and curtains during examinations, procedures and interviews.
- Provide a robe or second gown to ambulating patients and cover patients being transported.
- Make sure gowns are the right size for patients.
- Affirm patients' rights to make choices regarding their care.

Beaumont®
William Beaumont Hospital

Used with permission from William Beaumont Hospital, Troy, Michigan.

Appendix 8.8 William Beaumont Hospital's Performance Standards Commitment

William Beaumont Hospital
Troy

Performance Standards Commitment
William Beaumont Hospital, Troy

I have read and understand the Performance Standards that were developed by William Beaumont Hospital, Troy employees, and understand they are a measure of work performance. They are printed on cards to be attached to my identification badge and were attached to this document.

I understand by incorporating these standards as a measure of work performance, William Beaumont Hospital leadership makes it clear that we are all accountable for adhering to and practicing these standards.

I further understand that these standards apply equally to the interactions between all customer groups – patients, families, physicians and each other.

As a member of the William Beaumont Hospital, Troy Team, I am committed to the Standards and agree to not only hold myself accountable for doing so, but also to expect the same from all other Beaumont staff.

_____

Employee Signature

_____

Employee Name *(Please print)*   **ID #**

_____

Department

_____

Date

Used with permission from William Beaumont Hospital, Troy, Michigan.

Appendix 8.9 Baptist Health Care's WOW Card

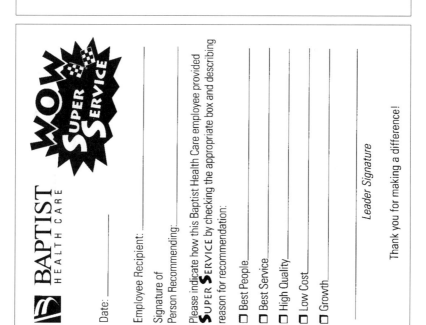

Living the values and **Exceeding** the Standards to **Achieve** our vision of making Baptist Health Care the **Best** health system in America.

The mission of Baptist Health Care is to provide superior service based on Christian values to improve the quality of life for people and communities served.

Attitude
Appearance
Communication
Call Lights
Commitment to Co-Workers
Customer Waiting
Elevator Etiquette
Privacy
Safety Awareness
Sense of Ownership

BAPTIST HEALTH CARE

BAPTIST HEALTH CARE

WOW SUPER SERVICE

Date: _____

Employee Recipient: _____

Signature of
Person Recommending: _____

Please indicate how this Baptist Health Care employee provided **S**UPER **S**ERVICE by checking the appropriate box and describing reason for recommendation:

☐ Best People _____
☐ Best Service _____
☐ High Quality _____
☐ Low Cost _____
☐ Growth _____

_____
Leader Signature

Thank you for making a difference!

Used with permission from Baptist Health Care Corporation, Pensacola, Florida.

Appendix 8.10 Bristol Hospital's WOW Certificate

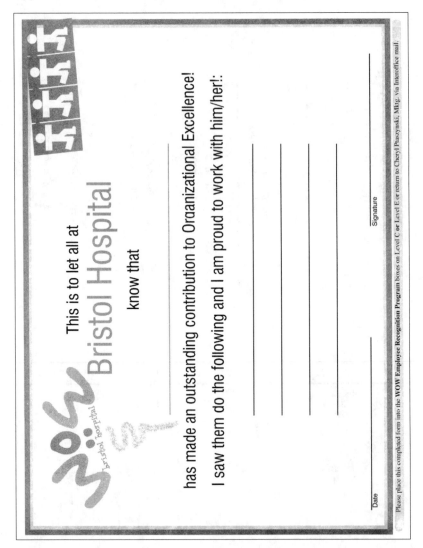

Used with permission from Bristol Hospital, Connecticut

Appendix 8.11 Kern Medical Center's Tell-A-Gram

Tell-A-Gram
a great way to say thank you

9997-3075 (4/99)

Recipient: _First and Last Name (One card per person or department)_ _____

Name of Department: _____

Date Service Performed: _____

Time Observed: _____

This person has provided outstanding customer service in the following way:

_____
_____
_____
_____
_____
_____
_____
_____

Please print your name and telephone number (required).

Name _____ Phone _____

Tell-A-Gram

The Tell-A-Gram acknowledges a special act of customer service. It is an expression of "going the extra mile".

Have you seen an employee(s) or department demonstrate a special act of service toward a customer or co-worker? Has someone done something to make your time pleasant or comfortable? Has a co-worker helped to make your job a little bit easier?

If the answer is yes, please acknowledge this example of commitment to outstanding customer service by giving that person (or department) a Tell-A-Gram.

Anyone may give a Tell-A-Gram - patient, customer, volunteer, employee, vendor, visitor, or guest.

Simply fill out the reverse side of this card and briefly describe the special act which deserves recognition. Then, place the card in the specially designated Tell-A-Gram boxes or mail to:

KMC Human Resources
1830 Flower Street
Bakersfield, CA 93305

We will make sure the Tell-A-Gram is delivered to the person, their supervisor and the Customer Service Task Force.

Thank you for your participation!

KERN MEDICAL CENTER

Used with permission from Kern Medical Center, Bakersfield, California.

CHAPTER 9

The Emergency Department: A Special Case

PATIENT SATISFACTION IN the ED offers special challenges. The emergency encounter is brief (relatively speaking) and usually stressful. Establishing rapport is difficult. For many patients, the ED visit is their first experience with the hospital or medical center and its related services. This means that patients' ED experience has major marketing implications. You may not be making a buck on the ED, but if patients decide they don't like your emergency facilities, you'll soon find your more profitable service revenues falling! Finally, patient and staff views of "emergency" may differ significantly. The nature of the emergency patient constituency is changing, and staff are frequently unprepared to face this new healthcare customer.

ARE THEY PATIENTS OR CUSTOMERS?

Caring, dedicated staff often have difficulty viewing patients as customers, yet the shifting nature of hospital care demands precisely such a perspective. As hospitals expand the range of services they offer (to attract managed care contracts as well as patients in general), brand naming becomes important. Each year, 20,000 to 70,000 patients pass through an ED. If patients are turned off by the experience, they may opt not to use the hospital's OR, or physician practice (or birthing center or cardiac center or home health agency) later on. The opposite is true, too. If patients are highly satisfied with emergency care, positive marketing has occurred. They will be more likely to select the hospital or its affiliated services for future care needs. Moreover, up to half of all inpatients are admitted through the ED. If satisfied with the emergency experience, they enter the hospital more positively predisposed toward inpatient care. This positive predisposition translates into greater collaboration and less likelihood of claims.

Do patients view themselves as customers?

We were surprised (as were Press, Ganey's emergency survey clients) to discover that the item most highly correlated with the likelihood of patients recommending the ED to others is not a technical quality issue. Rather, it's the issue of value. *Of all items on the emergency survey, the one most highly related to satisfaction was "emergency care was worth the money charged."*

Patients increasingly recognize that they are customers. Through insurance premiums, salary reductions, or co-pays, the majority are paying for emergency care one way or another, and they know it. They pay for everything else in their lives and have come to expect and demand both service and value.

Thom Mayer, chief ED physician at Inova Fairfax Hospital (Falls Church, Virginia), says they're both patients and customers. Some are almost all patient and more "horizontal" (very sick and very "out of it"). Some are mostly customer and conceptually more "vertical" (minimally sick, ambulatory, maximally aware of what's going on). Every patient is to some extent a customer (Mayer and Cates 1998):

A young mother (with insurance) brings her baby into the ED, stating that she accidentally spilled hot tea on her child's arm. Seeing only a slight bit of redness, the triage nurse makes the woman wait. Finally seen by a doctor, she is told that "there's nothing there" and that she "can put some salve on the baby's arm when you get home."

"What salve?" she asks. "Any one you have at home," answers the doctor curtly.

The mother leaves very upset. She angrily says, "My baby's arm is burned. After all this time waiting I'm only told to go home and put some salve on it? Any old salve! Maybe I have some salve at home and maybe I don't! What kind of treatment is this?" Here, she feels that her baby has received insufficient and rather cavalier care. She is unaware, of course, that it takes just as much medical expertise to judge that nothing is wrong as to diagnose a real problem. She leaves feeling she hasn't gotten value for her money. She wants medical care. But she's clearly very much a customer for this care.

Mothers who bring their children into the ED are always 100 percent customer and 0 percent patient.

Here is a positive example of a patient getting her money's worth.

A 30-something woman presents with a complaint of having "burned my mouth while eating ice cream. I took a big bite and a huge glob of it stuck to the roof of my mouth." She feels somewhat embarrassed by the incident. The physician examines her and tells her that she must gargle with salt water every two hours for the remainder of the day. "Don't miss a single time," he admonishes. She leaves very satisfied. The doctor has taken her seriously and made her feel that her decision to come to *this* ED was proper.

Both of these women were a small percent patient and a large percent customer.

When my company switched insurance plans because of some employees' dissatisfaction with our PPO's network hospital, it was largely ED experiences that triggered the defection. Now our growing staff use the emergency department, outpatient clinics, physician practices, and inpatient facilities of the competing hospital. Did the first hospital lose patients or customers?

WHO IS AN EMERGENCY PATIENT?

Many patients "shouldn't" be in the emergency department. Just ask your staff! Staff have yet to come to grips with the fact that perhaps half the patients are using the ED for primary care, rather than strict emergencies. The U.S. government estimates that close to 55 percent of ED patients are nonurgent (McCaig 1994). A typical ED staff estimates this at closer to 75 percent.

The problem with categorizing patients as "primary care" versus "real emergency" lies with the definition and—more precisely—*whose* perspective is driving the definition. A new mother presents with her baby at 2 in the afternoon, stating that her baby "didn't eat lunch." Staff eyes roll. Another "crock" is here "wasting our time." It's a good bet that she'll be punished (for presenting "inappropriately") by being made to wait. If a researcher subsequently were to use the medical records to do a study of ED use by emergent versus primary care patients, the young mother would surely be defined as a "primary care" case. To her, however, her problem is an emergency and staff do not seem to be taking her very seriously. She is still insecure with the responsibilities of motherhood and is frightened by the change in her new infant's eating pattern. To her, it's an emergency.

This can lead highly trained emergency professionals to feel "abused" by patients, especially during busy shifts. How easy is it to satisfy customers you feel are abusing you?

WHAT IS AN "EMERGENCY"?

In a previous chapter we discussed patients and staff as representing two different cultures. This is certainly the case in the ED.

Differences in values and expectations begin with the very definition of "emergency" and the proper function of the emergency department. To staff, the ED's function is essentially to stabilize patients. To patients, the function is to *heal,* not merely to stabilize. Thus, the emergency encounter often begins with significant misunderstanding of its very purpose. What constitutes an "emergency" in the first place? Patients define a medical problem as an emergency when one or more of three thresholds are crossed:

a. *Threshold of discomfort:* The pain or discomfort is at an unbearable level.
b. *Threshold of anxiety:* The condition causes such anxiety that the patient feels compelled to seek professional opinions and/or help.
c. *Threshold of inconvenience:* The condition interferes with valued behaviors or activities.

All of these are relative and variable. *Discomfort* can be immediate, intense, and unbearable, or it can become unbearable after hours or days have passed. "Why didn't you come right after you fell down?" inquires the doctor, rather exasperated. "It didn't hurt so much then," replies the patient, "and I could move it, so I figured it was only a sprain, not a break." Here, low initial pain, interpreted through a specific EM or explanatory model ("if it don't hurt, it ain't broke") kept the patient from coming to the ED in a timely manner. The doctor's exasperation, however, is surely communicated to the patient, who is made to feel he has done something wrong.

Anxiety is in the eye of the anxious one. For many people, vomiting or urinating bright red blood would likely create sufficient anxiety to spur a quick trip to the ED. A deep nasty gash could trigger the same. But anything could trigger anxiety. The mother bringing her baby in at 2 in the afternoon because the child didn't eat lunch has reached her own anxiety threshold. So too had the man who was finally frightened enough after 36 hours of mild but constant chest pain. From the staff perspective, the woman "shouldn't" have become anxious because her baby had not eaten lunch. The fellow with the chest pain should have become anxious a whole lot sooner. Yet to him, not the pain but its persistence triggered the decision to seek emergency treatment. In both cases, staff feel frustration and this frustration can be perceived by patients. Staff believe that their job is to treat "real" sickness or accident, and to do so in a timely manner. Patients are often perceived as thwarting these efforts.

Inconvenience is typically viewed as an illegitimate justification for postponing treatment or for coming to the ED in the first place. A woman comes in with an ankle sprain that occurred three or four days earlier. She has four children who must be driven to school daily. She participates in a rotating car pool with friends and neighbors. The sprain now prevents her from stepping on the brake pedal with force and she fears this will prevent her from fulfilling her driving obligations for the other car pool parents. A young man comes in with a three-day-old problem because tomorrow he must leave for reserve army duty. A young woman comes in with a cough she's had for days. She comes in now because she leaves on a vacation at 6 the next morning. She has a regular physician, but his office won't open till 9 AM.

Almost all ED visits reflect some social, economic, or other "nonmedical" component. An elderly woman drags her husband into the ED to "have his heart examined." She claims that he's been acting strangely lately, been out of breath, and may be having a heart attack. He denies feeling sick. She has demanded that he "come to the emergency room to settle this once and for all!" It's a power struggle as much as it's a medical event.

A middle-aged man brings his boss into the ED. He has insisted the boss accompany him to prove to his boss that he really is sick and really should be excused from work (with sick pay, of course). The motive for the visit is economic as well as medical.

When patients such as these come to the ED for "official proof" of sickness, staff may become frustrated. This is not a "proper" reason for seeking emergency care and tying up the time of busy professionals. Resentment of patients can be a result.

THE "DOUBLE BIND"

In all of these instances, staff feel beleaguered by patients who should not have come in the first place or who should have come at a more appropriate time. To many ED staff, patients should know *what* is appropriate to bring to the ED for treatment, and *when* it's appropriate to bring it. Of course, once in the ED, patients should shut up and offer concise information only—not opinions or diagnoses or treatment suggestions of their own. In this way, patients are put in a double bind, an uncomfortable situation in which they are punished for (on the one hand) not knowing medicine and (on the other hand) for audaciously claiming to know some medicine by requesting specific treatment.

> Why didn't you come in earlier?" exclaims the nurse to a 40-year-old white professional-looking male who presents around midnight with a deep, encrusted gash over his eye. The cut had occurred early that same morning. "I had a lot to do, and it stopped bleeding, so I figured it could wait till I had time," the patient explains. " I came in for some stitches. Can you minimize the scarring?" The nurse is frustrated by this patient, and testily replies: "No, we can't just "sew it up" like that and make it look nice! It's dried completely open. Now it has to be cleaned out and that won't be fun, and you'll probably have a much more obvious scar than if you'd come in sooner!

Here she verbally punishes the patient for both presenting at the wrong time and daring to suggest the course of treatment.

> A 35-year-old middle-class white woman presents with a sore throat. "I'm leaving on vacation tomorrow," she adds, "and I know exactly

what I need to get rid of it." She tells the triage nurse that she has had this same kind of sore throat before, and that a specific, named antibiotic always cures it quickly. She simply wants a prescription. She is assigned to a treatment cubicle and waits. Another nurse comes in to take a preliminary history and is given the same request. The frustrated patient waits even longer until a physician comes in. She reiterates her familiarity with the type of sore throat ("I've had this half a dozen times before") and requests the specific antibiotic. "This antibiotic always hits the sore throat fast. I've got to leave tomorrow morning and I need this now to knock it out so I can enjoy the vacation." The physician demurs, tells her he's calling for lab tests consisting of a throat culture and a blood analysis. Upon hearing of the blood test, the woman is now even more frustrated. The physician informs her that she may be suffering from anemia. The woman is furious over the fact that the physician has not taken her sore throat ideas seriously, and has further inserted a totally unexpected explanatory model (anemia) into the interaction. She ultimately gets a prescription for the very antibiotic she wants but leaves extremely dissatisfied with the ED. "She thinks she's the doctor," comments the physician, "and then she demands special treatment just because she's going on vacation to enjoy herself tomorrow." During the entire interaction, the doctor was coolly professional.

Harried ED staff may overlook the fact that the patient "has a life," in addition to a cough, pain, or gash. In chapter 3, we discussed the importance of the various roles that define each person's life and identity. These roles are brought to the ED, just as they are brought to the physician's office or hospital bed. Even before patients come to the ED, their various roles and identities interact with the physical problem to enhance or retard time-appropriate health-seeking behavior. It is precisely because these roles define our lives that we seek treatment when we are sick. We want to resume the roles, identities, and activities disrupted by the problem. All patients bring their threatened identities with them to the ED. Thus, staff must be sensitive to patients' reasons for coming in *now*. The question "why didn't you come in sooner?" is essentially irrelevant. Knowing what is presently bothering the patient enough to trigger an ED visit can help staff establish quick rapport and design a treatment regimen that is more likely to be followed. The woman leaving for vacation tomorrow morning will likely not follow a recommendation of "several days' bed rest." Moreover, her travels may make it difficult or inconvenient for her to take medication three or four times daily. Here, a once-a-day medication will more likely result in compliance.

TAKING PATIENTS SERIOUSLY

This is what it boils down to, really: for whatever reason, patients have decided to define their problem as an emergency and bring it to your hospital. In a number of ways staff can demonstrate that they do—or do not—take these patients seriously. Patients want to be greeted by someone who knows enough emergency medicine to appreciate their problem. Patients want to be admitted to the treatment area quickly. They do not want to be shunted aside to an obvious "urgent care" or "fast-track" area that effectively tells them their claim to be an emergency patient is not taken seriously by staff. Press, Ganey's national data shows a modest yet clear dip in satisfaction for patients in EDs with a separate on-site facility for non-urgent patients.

Not that a fast-track facility in the ED automatically generates lower satisfaction; perhaps it should not be too obviously identifiable. Fast track could be a separate process, rather than a clearly separate place.

Patients come to the ED loaded with all of the cultural baggage we discussed in chapter 3. They have sifted through symptoms and decided which were relevant. They have sifted through their own and their friends' and family's explanations about what they've got and what should be done (their EMs). To a lesser or greater degree, the problem affects them emotionally. To some extent it has disrupted or threatened important roles and identities. The problem may also have shunted them into a sick role that they've successfully acted out at home and will act out in the ED. All of this is brought *with* the physical problem. Staff responses to these issues affect the patient's evaluation of care.

> A sixty-year-old white male presents with his wife, complaining about a swollen, sore foot. He repeatedly asks the nurse, and subsequently the physician, whether he shouldn't be prescribed a "footbath"—something like Epsom salts—in which to soak his swollen foot. The physician ignores the request, explaining that the man's problem is internal, not external. An antibiotic is prescribed and the physician leaves. The patient and wife are both vocally upset. To them, an "external" problem such as a swollen foot should be treated with an external solution.

Note that the couple do not view the swelling as a symptom, rather, it's the problem. Their EM results in dissatisfaction when the physician ignores their very clear concerns. He didn't take them seriously and they knew it.

MORAL EVALUATION OF PATIENTS

In a seminal study of ED staff attitudes toward patients, Roth and Douglas (1983) note that staff have a pretty clear idea of who is an "appropriate" patient. Good patients present at the proper time with problems that are truly emergent. They are grateful for treatment. They cooperate. They answer questions concisely and produce relevant information. They're not demanding or complaining. They tolerate discomfort "like adults" and try not to make noise that could upset other patients. They do not pretend to know as much medicine as the doctors. Ideally, in fact, they know nothing but their symptoms, which are presented clearly and accurately. They do not conjecture about causes or cures. Friends and relatives who accompany "good" patients comport themselves with calm, dignity, appreciation, and understanding about delays and treatment protocols.

In addition, "good" patients present with "proper" problems. Not only are they emergent, but they are ideally not the patient's fault (Becker et al. 1961, 322). Nor are their medical problems caused by disreputable activities (fights, unsafe sex, or dangerous acts such as motorcycling or in-line skating). A good patient did not acquire the problem nor present to the emergency staff while under the influence of alcohol or drugs. A good mother does not let her child get at poisonous substances under the kitchen sink. A good patient pays for care in one way or another and is not a freeloader.

Patients share many values with medical staff. They themselves may find their problems embarrassing or deserving of disdain.

An 80-year-old man presents at the ED complaining that he "lost consciousness" and fell on the sidewalk. He banged his head and wants it attended to. The physician suspects the patient may have suffered a stroke, and orders appropriate tests. The old man converses with a volunteer, confiding that he really didn't lose consciousness ("Well, yes, I really did, but after I fell"). Rather shamefacedly, he admits that he fell while attempting to kick a can that was lying on the sidewalk. "It was a childish thing to do," he says. He didn't tell the doctor because he "felt ashamed to be so stupid." Here, the patient brings his dignity with him to the ED and it results in a lie to the physician.

The point is that patients—anticipating (deservedly or not) disdain or ridicule—may lie to staff or attempt to mislead them. Given the brief one-shot nature of the emergency encounter, accurate histories must be elicited and cooperation encouraged. Thus, staff attitudes toward patients must support the goals of emergency treatment. This is accomplished when staff attitudes are observably caring, supportive and sympathetic. By "observably," we mean that tone of voice, body language, and actions demonstrate a clear, caring attitude.

Professional ED staff are largely middle class or above. Like patients, staff cannot leave their roles, identities, values, and prejudices at home. Drunks are disliked and treated coldly. "Frequent flyers" are the butts of jokes and made to wait. Fifteen-year-old single mothers are viewed with distaste (as well as with sorrow or disgust). Medicaid patients are often perceived as "freeloaders" and disdained. I have heard Medicaid patients referred to by staff as "gold-carders"—a judgmental reference to the fact that these patients can get good care without having to pay. I have also heard ED physicians talk of a "brown alert," when a particularly high number of Medicaid patients were present. Brown is the color of feces. Of course, this could not happen in *your* emergency department, but it happens in some. For whatever reason, it is not unusual for Medicaid patients to spend more time waiting than do privately insured patients.

I have come across all of these as causes for staff resentment of various types of patients. We're not talking about all emergency staff, or even most. But all staff are human and cannot avoid frustration with some patients at some time. These frustrations can affect staff judgements of the legitimacy of patient claims to emergency status and proper emergency treatment. Treatment will indeed be given, but the patient (customer) may pay a price.

Roth and Douglas (1983) find that staff may attempt to punish patients who offend their sense of moral propriety or offend their professional status by presenting with unworthy problems. Punishment takes various forms. Patients may be made to wait, they may not be looked in on by nurses. Interaction may be cool and professional but not friendly or comforting, or patients may be labeled.

LABELING

Verbal labels may be generic or patient specific. The disheveled guy with the torn shirt that looks like a cape may be referred to as "superman." The young man whimpering as his knife-fight wound is stitched may be denigrated as "Mr. Macho." More generically, the woman with vague stomach symptoms but no test-revealed pathology may be a "crock." The guy who has been to the ED three times in the past four weeks is a "frequent flyer." I came across an ED where drunks, druggies, and patients with vague, untreatable symptoms were referred to as "oids" (as in "humanoids"). Most "oids" were Medicaid patients. In yet another ED, staff would refer to similar patients as "3-footers," "4-footers," or "5-footers" (referring to turkey wing span. A "5-footer" was a real turkey!).

Patients' moral legitimacy (as well as their legitimacy as ED patients) may also be judged and labeled by staff. The 14-year-old girl presenting with low stomach pains may be referred to as a "crotch case" and assumed to be suffering from a sexually transmitted disease. I saw one such child being asked if she were taking any medication. She responded by saying that she was taking birth control pills. Staff asked for the pill dispenser and taped it to her chart, which was hung on the chart board in full view of everyone on both sides of the counter. One of Press, Ganey's employees recalls the following incident at a local ED:

> I was in the emergency room for something and I was waiting to see the doctor. I could hear him talking to a patient in the bed next to me on the other side of the curtain. She was a young black girl, about 14 or so, and had come in complaining about stomach pains. Her mother was with her. The doctor asks the girl, "are you sexually active?"
>
> Can you believe that? Right in front of her mother, he asks her that! How embarrassing for the girl!

Here, the physician may be responding to what he believes to be immoral behavior by confronting (punishing) the girl about her sexuality directly in front of her mother. The physician also may have been reflecting his personal stereotypes about blacks and their sexual behavior. The net result, however, is that a moral judgement was made and the patient punished. As a side issue, the comments were overheard by another patient, who was also turned off by the interaction. Walls are thin in EDs. I have seen nurses (standing just outside the curtain) purposely and loudly discussing a mother's ability to care for her child (her baby was in for ingesting some household cleaner kept under the sink). Their comments were designed to punish.

Labeling need not be verbal. Patients who are viewed as behavioral problems or disdained for one reason or another may be assigned to "room 11." Every ED has a "room 11" that is usually at a distance from the nursing station and to which are assigned "sensitive" patients (such as rape victims) or, more usually, disreputable or unruly patients, or teenage girls with vague stomach pains or obvious STDs. Even if placed in a standard treatment room, a disdained patient may receive minimal visits from nurses and cool interaction from physicians. Recall chapter 3's discussion about the effect of labeling on staff interaction with patients.

DELAYS AND WAITING TIME

In the past few years there have been dozens of conferences on reducing ED delays. What, however, is a "delay"? Do we count total time spent in the ED? Or only time spent in a waiting room outside the treatment area? Or time spent waiting in a treatment cubicle? And are we talking about *real* time or *perceived* time?

People talk about getting patients in and out in less than 30 minutes. Is this realistic? Is it even desirable? Dr. Jim Espinosa, head of the emergency department of Overlook Hospital in Summit, New Jersey, reports that ED satisfaction scores rose as total time decreased. That is, until patients began spending an average of less than 30 minutes in the ED. At that point, satisfaction scores started falling again. Espinosa believes the decline was because patients began to feel that their examination and treatment was rushed and not thorough.

Figure 9.1 shows the distribution of total time patients spend in the ED. These and subsequent data are from the current Press, Ganey

Figure 9.1 Total Time Spent in the ED

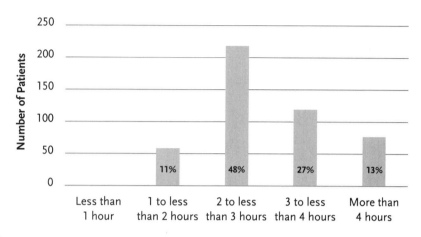

Source: Press, Ganey database. 2002.

database, and represent responses from over 800,000 patients treated at over 500 emergency departments across the country. Close to 90 percent of all patients report spending two or more hours in the ED. Expecting to readily reduce stays to an hour (let alone a half hour or less) may be unrealistic for the majority of patients.

By and large, the longer patients are in the ED, the less satisfied they are with overall care (Figure 9.2). Very few patients (only 16 percent) spend more than four total hours in the average emergency department. They also tend to be sicker and typically require a longer period of observation or treatment. After the forth hour, satisfaction drops by a modest 2 to 3 points hourly. During the initial four hours, however, satisfaction drops by 4 points per hour. This suggests that if you want to reduce total ED time and improve satisfaction, focus on getting the less acute patients out faster.

How much of the total time spent in the ED constitutes a "delay"? And what is a "delay"?

Figure 9.2 Likelihood of Recommending the ED by Hours Spent in the ED

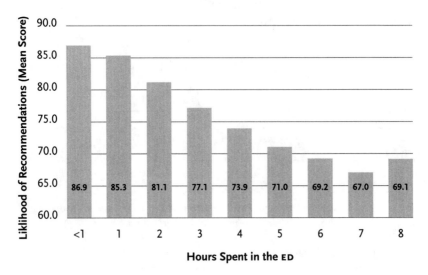

Source: Press, Ganey database. 2002.

Consider the following typical patient experience:

1. Arrival.
2. Interview with admitting personnel.
3. Triage (if triage nurse is not doing the admitting).
4. Possible wait in external waiting room if ED is busy.
5. Admission to treatment area.
6. Nurse takes vitals and information.
7. Physician visits—may treat or call for tests.
8. Technologist or nurse takes blood, EKG, etc.
9. Possible trip to x-ray.
10. X-ray taken.
11. Wait for escort back to ED treatment room.
12. Physician returns with results. Discusses. Explains, treats, or prescribes.

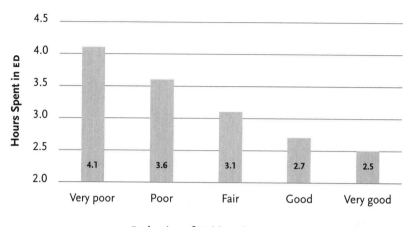

Evaluation of Waiting Time to See Doctor

13. Nurse "closes." Discharge or slated for admission to inpatient bed.
14. (If necessary) Wait for transport upstairs.

This sequence is pretty typical and logical, but not for the patient. The patient cannot predict these events. Between each event is a potential delay while the patient waits for an unknown someone to do an unknown something. The typical patient experiences at least 8 or 9 of these events, and as many as all 14. There may be at least two waits for the doctor.

Most patients spend little or no time in the lobby waiting area; almost all the time is spent back in the treatment area. Patients view the entire time in the treatment area as "treatment time." Until they leave the ED, "treatment" is not over, so, until they are discharged, they are theoretically waiting to be treated.

Figure 9.4 Likelihood of Recommending ED

Likelihood Correlated with:	Actual Waiting Time	Waiting Room Wait	Treatment Wait	Informed About Delays
	−.160	.592	.648	.732

Note: All correlations are significant at the .000 level.

Because the physician is the key person who diagnoses, treats, and releases them, patients equate total time in the ED with time spent waiting for the physician to treat them.

Figure 9.3 illustrates total time spent in the ED and its effect on patients' judgements of the appropriateness of the time spent waiting for the physician. Given our discussion above, we view the "wait for the physician" as equivalent to the patient's judging appropriateness of the total time spent in the treatment area. Clearly, as *most* of the patient's time is spent in the treatment area, the less time spent there, the more the patient views this time as appropriate.

It's important to note that those patients who are very satisfied with the time spent in the treatment area are still spending an average of 2½ total hours in the ED, therefore, reducing time is not in itself the key to satisfaction with emergency care. The best method of gauging the effect of delays on patients is via satisfaction surveys, not time logs by staff.

We must be very careful to distinguish between total actual time spent in the ED and patients' judgements of the appropriateness of this time. The correlations in Figure 9.4 are most revealing: Patient satisfaction with the overall ED experience is definitely affected by judgements of the *appropriateness* of time spent in the waiting room and in the treatment area. Correlations of .592 and .648 are quite high. Not surprisingly, patients view time in the treatment area as somewhat more important than time in the external waiting room.

Figure 9.5 Rating of Satisfaction Correlated with Wait to See the Physician by Hours in ED and Information About Delays

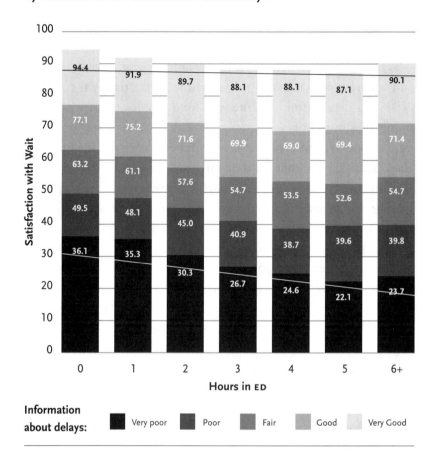

Far more interesting, however, is the correlation of "How well you were informed about delays?" with overall satisfaction. A correlation of .732 is very high. What it tells us is that *when patients are given information about what to expect, when to expect it, and why it didn't happen when expected, they are far more satisfied with the overall ED experience.*

The importance of explaining events and delays is strikingly exhibited in the rather formidable graph in Figure 9.5.

We've already looked at the relationship between total time in the ED and patient judgements of the appropriateness of the wait to see the physician. The longer the total time, the lower the satisfaction with the wait. But what if patients are given explanations about what is happening and why it's taking so long?

The darkest bars reflect very poor information about delays—and very low satisfaction with the wait to be treated by the doctor. Note that satisfaction with the wait for a physician drops about 13 points—from 36 to 23 (on a 100-point scale)—as the hours pass. The lightest bars are quite different. They reflect very good information about delays. Note that for the same total time spent, patients rate the wait to be treated *60 to 70 points higher* than when poor information about delays is given. Moreover, with the passing of hours, the drop in satisfaction is small—less than 7 points. What this shows, again, is that information and perception of appropriateness of time underlie satisfaction, not actual hours spent in the ED. *The more information given about what is happening, the more that patients view the passing time as acceptable.*

Resetting the Clock

One of our client EDs noted low scores in waiting time. They solved the problem simply. Anyone who has contact with the patient—from admitting clerk to nurse to doctor to lab tech to whoever—is responsible for telling the patient what will happen next, who will do it, and approximately when it will happen. Overestimating the time until the next event is preferable to underestimating it. Whenever the doctor or nurse enters the treatment cubicle, they apologize for any delay. The results have been remarkable. Satisfaction with overall care has escalated, as has satisfaction with the time spent in the treatment area.

The patient's clock starts ticking the moment he or she is admitted, and keeps on ticking throughout the whole treatment. However, if patients are given new information about when the next

Figure 9.6 Issues Correlated with Likelihood of Recommending ED

	Correlation Coefficient
Degree to which your emergency room care was worth the money charged	0.85
Degree to which staff cared about you as a person	0.81
How well you were kept informed about delays you may have experienced in the emergency room	0.74
Amount of attention the nurses paid to you	0.70
Nurses' concern to keep you informed about your treatment	0.70
Staff concern to keep family/friends informed about your treatment or condition	0.69
Degree to which nurses took your problems seriously	0.68
Courtesy with which family/friends were treated	0.68
Doctor's concern for your comfort while treating you	0.67
Degree to which the doctor took your problems seriously	0.67
Doctor's concern to explain tests and treatments	0.66
Waiting time in the treatment area before you were seen by a doctor	0.65
Technical skill of the nurses	0.65
Nurses' concern for your privacy	0.64
Courtesy of the nurses	0.64
Courtesy of the doctor	0.64
Advice you were given by the doctor about caring for yourself at home or obtaining follow-up medical care	0.64
Waiting time before you were brought into the treatment area	0.60
Staff concern to let family and friends be with you while you were being treated	0.59
Comfort of the registration waiting room	0.57
Courtesy of the person who took your blood	0.53
Helpfulness of the person at the registration desk	0.52
Privacy you felt during the registration interview	0.50
How well your blood was taken (quickly, little pain, etc.)	0.49
How satisfactory was the process to obtain your insurance/billing information	0.49
Waiting time in the x-ray department	0.49
Courtesy of the x-ray technician	0.46
Convenience of parking	0.39

Notes: n=548 hospitals, n=841,412 patients

event will occur, they reset their clocks for that time ("It'll take about 20 minutes for me to analyze this blood and for the doctor to get back to you"). Otherwise, the only referent is the *entire* time spent from the moment of admission.

THE IDEAL EMERGENCY DEPARTMENT

More than anything, simply knowing what is important to patients offers a solution to the question of "how do we improve satisfaction with our ED?" Figure 9.6 presents a list correlating all items in the Press, Ganey ED satisfaction survey with "likelihood of recommending this emergency room to others." All items on the survey are significantly linked to satisfaction; however, those near the top of the list (with higher correlation coefficients) have a closer relationship to likelihood of recommending. By focusing attention on these issues, emergency departments can make significant improvements. Note that the majority of key items are interaction related. In their study of emergency department patient satisfaction, Hall and Press conclude:

> Large numbers (typically the majority) of emergency patients present with fairly simple problems (not necessarily to them, of course!). As they receive appropriately simple technical care (if any) and leave "stabilized" rather than "cured," it is not surprising that various studies (as well as ours) conclude that interpersonal factors may contribute most to satisfaction with the ED. (1996, 527)

Care in the ideal emergency department addresses these factors directly or indirectly. Following are general characteristics of an ideal emergency department—one in which concern for patient satisfaction drives all aspects of care, from physical plant to organization and interaction. We are not going to mention one obvious "ideal"— that the ED is big enough, modern enough, designed well enough and staffed well enough to make a positive impression on patients regardless of any organizational or behavioral characteristics. In truth, you do not need a modern facility to satisfy anxious, uncomfortable patients who want attention, empathy, reassurance, and appropriate treatment. Modern, cheerful facilities help reduce patient anxiety, but to increase patient satisfaction significantly, far more is needed.

1. *First and foremost, the ideal ED is self-aware.* Its staff recognize that departmental organization is cultural in nature, and riddled with ritual and justifications such as "we've always done it this way." The ideal ED approaches every rule, work habit, and protocol (that isn't specifically mandated by law or regulatory agencies) from a perspective of "zero-based budgeting." That is, each action must be justified by more than an appeal to tradition. In most EDs, for example, nursing notes are typically written out in narrative form. For most patient problems, however, a simple check-list format might work well. This reduces time spent documenting common presenting symptoms, health history, and so forth.

Union Hospital in Union, New Jersey demonstrated zero-based budgeting when it redesigned its triage process. Standing orders were written for many common ailments such as abdominal pain, ankle injuries, and others. The triage nurse can initiate a set of standing x-ray protocols, order a CBC or other routine blood work and initiate an IV. Thus, patients perceive that they are being taken seriously and much time is also saved. In this case, it was decided that many routine aspects of diagnosis or treatment did not demand a physician's time.

Overlook Hospital, in Summit, New Jersey decided that the "need" to have all x-rays assessed by a radiology specialist prior to delivery of the film to the emergency physician was a time-consuming ritual that could be abolished. Films were already delivered directly to the ED docs during evenings and weekends. According to literature research, emergency physicians had been determined to be quite capable of accurately recognizing whether a problem was visible in the x-ray. Overlook Hospital subsequently standardized this practice for all shifts.

Lourdes Hospital in Binghamton, New York, uses the same procedure, but also has a radiologist look at all films within two hours and report back to the ED physician if there is any difference in interpretation.

2. *The ideal ED has some provision for fast-track treatment that appears (to the patient) to be part of the ordinary ED process.* Thus, many non-acute patients can be seen more quickly without being made to feel that their problem is not taken seriously. Fast-track areas could be staffed with RNs and physician assistants (PAs), but patients will likely be more satisfied if a "real doctor" makes even a brief appearance.

3. *Everyone in the ideal ED thinks entrepreneurially.* All recognize that patients are also customers and have economic value to the broader medical center network. To legitimize this orientation, both the CEO and CFO have both led workshops attended by all ED staff (especially physicians), informing them of the economic importance to the entire institution of an entrepreneurially oriented emergency department. In addition, attendance at a customer service workshop is mandated (again, this mandate includes physicians).

4. *Everyone, from receptionists to physicians, knows the ED's latest satisfaction scores.* Patient satisfaction is a permanent agenda item at department meetings, and physicians are required to attend.

5. *If the emergency physicians belong to a practice management group, their contract with the hospital puts the group at risk for some compensation reduction if patient satisfaction scores fall below a target number.* At the same time, the hospital is committed to providing additional compensation if satisfaction levels exceed the target.

6. *Group discussions are organized and managed by a facilitator who can lead staff to confront their feelings about who is or is not a "legitimate" emergency patient.* Discussion deals with issues of moral evaluation as well as medical evaluation of "deserving" patients. Discussion also confronts the potential effect of staff "attitudes" on their interaction with and management of patients. Staff may also need to confront elements of racism and other socioeconomic prejudices that can affect labeling of and interaction with patients.

7. *The admitting desk is situated in such a manner as to maximize the potential for privacy.*

8. *Admitting is done by an RN, not a clerk.* If a clerk is hired, however, she is empathetic and knowledgeable, and is mature in both manner and appearance (particularly if not an RN), thus fostering trust in his or her ability to understand the problem or take it seriously. Many people are uncomfortable or embarrassed telling very personal things to someone who looks relatively young and/or who does not appear to be a nurse or physician. Ideally, the admitting person is the triage nurse.

9. *Bedside registration is the rule.* The patient is ushered into the treatment area before financial or other registration information is elicited. This says, "Your problem is taken more seriously than your insurance status."

10. *Patients cannot see into one another's rooms.* They are asked if they want their door or curtain closed or left open (so they can see the staff and be distracted by the action).

11. *Every person who contacts the patient explains what's going to happen next, who will do it, and when it will occur.* Every person who subsequently interacts with the patient does the same. Staff who have been delayed apologize to the patient.

12. *The patient is offered a blanket, pillow, or other comfort-maker.* If appropriate, a soft drink or water and/or snack is offered.

13. *A chair or two are available in the treatment cubicle for visitors.* And there is a stool for the doctor to sit on, and a local phone, and a TV. A soft drink and snack machine are conveniently located out in the waiting room that takes tokens that are provided (at no cost) by the admitting desk.

14. *A nurse looks in on the patient frequently, asking if everything's OK*—and sounds like she sincerely wants to know.

15. *Friends and relatives who accompany the patient are treated in a friendly, courteous manner.* Staff demeanor communicates to guests that their presence is expected and welcomed, not merely tolerated.

16. *If the ED is a busy one, volunteer "patient liaisons" make the round of patients, keeping them company, chatting, performing small errands, explaining emergency room routine or "culture"* (why the delay, why the doctor hasn't come back yet; "why" that patient in the next cubicle is getting attention now when he came in *after* me, etc.).[1]

17. *The physician introduces himself or herself and sits so as to minimize intimidation.* The physician touches the patient, and chats for a second of two before getting down to business.

18. *The physician elicits the patient's "explanatory model" (EM).* Given the shortness of time, all that is required are two questions: "What do you think is the matter?" (obviously this can be omitted for a number of types of injuries), and "What do you think should be done?" Many patients will not respond or will say, "I don't know—you're the doctor." This happens a lot, but you have to ask. If patients respond, their EM is at least listened to and, where appropriate, accommodated. This encourages trust and empathy. It shows that the patient is taken seriously.

19. *The patient is asked why he or she is coming in* now, *if the problem occurred significantly earlier.* If at all possible, treatment protocols should reflect the patient's present need (social, recreational, emotional, whatever) for treatment. After telling patients how to care for themselves at home, physicians elicit some information about the patient's ability to comply with discharge instructions. Care regimens are adjusted accordingly. If post-ED care regimens conflict with accustomed living habits or special occasions, the result will often (if not usually) be noncompliance.

20. *Patients are not placed in a double-bind situation.* Staff do not expect them to know when it's appropriate to come in or what problems are appropriate for emergency treatment.

21. *Patients' emotions are expected and tolerated* (as long as they don't disrupt the ED or significantly affect other patients). Staff assume that patients may be suffering, scared, threatened, and embarrassed. This is an emergency room, not a bank lobby.

22. *Professional and social prejudices are hidden from patients.* Sexually active teens, overly worried mothers, frequent flyers, and overly demanding Medicaid patients have not come to the ED to be morally corrected or punished.

23. *Staff never discuss patients where they can be overheard.*

24. *Everyone (doctors, nurses, lab techs, therapists) explains what he or she is doing and why.*

25. *"Closing" is done by the physician, not a nurse.* Ideally, the doctor sits during the final statement and instructions. Usually this is the time for asking if the patient "has any questions." If the doctor's voice and body language say "I'm on my way out of here, make it fast," it is unlikely that the patient will ask anything. Such behavior also encourages non-compliance.

26. *Patients are phoned later in the evening after discharge by a nurse who asks how they are doing, if they have any questions and if they have followed through on the discharge instructions.* Union Hospital (New Jersey) does this, and the call is scripted to make it easier and faster. Very busy EDs may not be able to do this. Lourdes (Binghamton, New York) does not phone everyone, just those whose diagnoses represent conditions judged to create a risk for the patient. Patients with these diagnoses are phoned the next day. Patients who leave AMA (against medical advice) are also phoned.

These are but a few characteristics of the "ideal emergency department." The list could be much longer. Note that almost all elements require modest behavioral or attitudinal changes, rather than construction or major reorganization of tasks. Establishment of a fast-track service might be an exception, but even this could be managed with imaginative staffing changes using existing facilities. Every ED in the country already exhibits many of these "ideal" characteristics.

ONE EMERGENCY DEPARTMENT'S SUCCESS STORY

Overlook Hospital in Summit, New Jersey offers an example of what can be done. In their entry for Press, Ganey's national "Success Story" competition (1998), Jim Espinosa, M.D. (Overlook's emergency department's medical director), and Linda Kosnik, R.N. (the former ED nurse manager and current chief nursing officer), write:

> We need to have a systematic way to communicate with our customers. It is a sobering thought to realize that most of us do not ask our patients and other customers often enough what *they* think and feel about the service which we are providing. We assume that we know, and we all too often intuit incorrectly. A patient may be discharged from the ED with a perception that no one cared, and

might vow never to return. Yet the chart might reflect utter and complete fidelity to ED protocols. The performance to standards might have been excellent, but the perception might have been ruined by a noisy environment, or the busy and very aloof manner of a physician or nurse.

With patient satisfaction scores far lower than they wanted, Overlook's emergency department went to work. In the third quarter of 1996 a "Patient Satisfaction Summit" was held. Attendance was mandatory for all emergency physicians, nurses, technicians, secretaries, registrars, and volunteers.

Interdisciplinary work groups were formed and each was assigned a section of the satisfaction survey and charged with improving those aspects of care. Each work group had to:

- Review satisfaction data for their assigned survey section;
- Brainstorm root causes for areas of dissatisfaction;
- Brainstorm possible solutions; and
- Agree on priorities for solutions, based on the satisfaction data.

Work groups shared their discussions with each other and shared suggestions. "Quick wins" were identified so as to generate early enthusiasm.

> The overall theme seemed to be that we would commit ourselves to providing breakthrough levels of service for discharged patients. The group identified that historically, most of our resources had been directed at [ED patients admitted to the hospital]. We needed to resource the discharged patient population. (Espinosa and Kosnik 1998)

Based on specific low-scoring items on the patient satisfaction survey (noted in parentheses), they decided on the following priorities for action:

1. Create a fast track: rooms, counters, lights, staffing, supplies, protocols (reduce delays, reduce waiting time to treatment area, provide access to physician, increase resources for discharged patients).
2. Reduce x-ray cycle time (reduce delays).
3. Reduce registration cycle time (reduce delays).
4. Move toward bedside registration (increase privacy satisfaction, improve waiting time to treatment area, improve satisfaction with billing process).
5. Reduce arrival to treatment by physician cycle time (reduce waiting time for physician).
6. Reduce pharmacy cycle time (reduce delays).
7. Complete ongoing environmental/structural improvements (cheerfulness).
8. Create an ED facelift: new floors, wallpaper, wall bumpers, counters, nursing station, borders (cheerfulness).
9. Open four-bed observation suite: rooms, counters, lights, staffing, supplies, protocols, televisions, phones (provide comfort items, reduce delays, allow family and friends to be with patient).
10. Create pediatric treatment room: crib, supplies, carts, murals (provide comfort items, reduce delays, allow family and friends to be with patient). Complete improvements to waiting room: fish tank, children's corner, VCR with Disney tapes, new furniture, new floors (increase comfort of waiting room).
11. Increase privacy in registration area: soundproof dividers (increase privacy, improve registration).
12. Purchase and install new chart rack system: visual display of chart movement through treatment process (reduce delay items).
13. Promote more effective use of patient tracking system: multiple monitors and CPUs (reduce delays, provide information about delays, increase adequacy of information to family and friends).

14. Improve temperature control in ED (increase comfort).
15. Provide sitting stools in patient rooms to promote physician and nurse eye contact during interviews (practitioner interaction items in survey and staff care about patient as person).
16. Purchase new stretchers (provide comfort items in survey).
17. Order business cards for physicians and nurses to be given at discharge (provide information about treatment and home care, nurse and physician courtesy).
18. Supply improved patient discharge instructions (provide nurse and physician information about treatment and home care).
19. Buy three-dimensional anatomy models of common fast-track problems, for example, of the foot, ankle, and elbow, for patient instruction (provide nurse and physician information about treatment and home care).
20. Create new on-call systems (reduce delays).

When action targets had been identified, the next step was to build commitment to the improvement process. This called for a "cultural revolution" that they stimulated by:

1. Scheduling lectures by patient satisfaction experts.
2. Reviewing relevant literature. All ED staff were required to read selected publications.
3. Attending presentations by benchmark hospitals with track records of success. This included 200 hours of leadership visits and consultation with Holy Cross Hospital (Chicago), Hermann Hospital (Houston), and Harris-Methodist (Fort Worth).
4. Bringing in a Disney Institute Lecturer for ED staff and senior hospital management.
5. Engaging in discussions with survey vender about satisfaction enhancement.

The following processes were then implemented:

1. Feedback of survey results to physicians and nurses. Where individual physicians were scored particularly low by one of their patients (a 1 or 2 on a 5-point scale), a written response from the physician (to ED management) was required. Conversely, very positive individual patient feedback was shared and used as encouragement.
2. Mini-sessions on handling difficult situations and people. This would encourage courtesy, helpfulness, concern, and problem solving.
3. Contests and rewards to improve satisfaction. In one contest, physicians were pitted against nurses for highest scores; in another contest staff held a "satisfaction pool" to see who could most accurately predict the next quarter's satisfaction scores.
4. A patient satisfaction bulletin board on which were posted scores, graphs, solution story boards, and positive letters or comments from patients.
5. Phoning of patients who made significantly positive or negative comments on the survey.
6. Promotion of the philosophy of the "Disney attitude."

Overlook's emergency department scores soared over the next several years. Total ED time for patients dropped significantly as admitting, x-ray, and treatment times were cut. Total turnaround time for nonurgent patients (treated in the new fast-track mode) dropped from 120 minutes to 60. Time from admission to being seen by a physician dropped from 31 minutes to an average of 19 minutes. Scores rose dramatically for almost all interactive and informational issues as well.

Although Overlook spent some bucks, money was not the key to their success. Much was a result of process, protocol, and organizational change that took little additional out of the budget.

CONCLUSIONS

In two senses, the ED is the gateway to the hospital. On the one hand, many patients are admitted to the inpatient sector from the ED. The ED experience can predispose the patient positively or negatively to events and interactions that follow. On the other hand, for thousands of prospective customers (of the hospital and its associated services), the ED may be the initial marketing experience.

Most important, of course, is that for all who enter the ED, care must be provided in such as way as to maximize its effectiveness. Because the contact between emergency patient and staff is brief, intense, and to some extent unavoidably impersonal, special care must be taken in designing protocols for patient/staff interaction and for controlling the patient's experience in the facility. Attention to patient satisfaction can have a significant effect on patient management and outcome in this unique, intense, stress-laden context.

ACTION FOR SATISFACTION

1. Approach every rule, work habit, and protocol from the perspective of "zero-based budgeting."
2. Create a fast-track treatment that will not be noticeably different to the patient.
3. Think (and encourage staff to think) like an entrepreneur.
4. Post satisfaction scores.
5. Hold physicians accountable for satisfaction scores.
6. Conduct discussions about staff attitudes in interactions with and management of patients.
7. Position the admitting desk to maximize patient privacy and hire an RN to man the desk.
8. Implement bedside registration.
9. Provide privacy for each patient. Staff never discuss patients where they can be overheard.

10. Make it a part of standard procedure to communicate with patients about what will happen next, who will do it, and when it will occur.
11. Provide for the patient's comfort with extra pillows, blankets, snacks, chairs for visitors, phones, and so forth.
12. Make it possible for nurses to check in on patients frequently. Teach staff to respond to patients and their visitors in a friendly, sincere manner.
13. Create a "patient liaison" position to care for the nonclinical needs of patients.
14. Train physicians to increase patient satisfaction by sitting when in the patient's presence, chatting with the patient, eliciting and listening to the patient's explanatory model, and so forth.
15. Train staff to listen to the patient's reasoning for seeking treatment, respect patient's knowledge levels and emotional responses to illness, and hide prejudices.
16. Make it standard procedure that a patient's final instructions are given by a physician who allows time for questions.
17. Phone patients after care to follow up on discharge instructions and provide further explanation if necessary.

NOTE

1. Obviously the patient has to give consent for this, but most are more than happy to have someone to chat with. Obviously too, staffing is the major issue. You would want the "liaisons" during the busiest times—especially the 4 p.m. to midnight shift. Liaisons can be standard volunteers or employees. Here's another idea: I started programs in two local emergency departments in South Bend almost 20 years ago and they are still running strong. Contact the social science departments at a local college or university (anthropology, sociology, psychology, economics; also try philosophy and theology). Ask if anyone is teaching a course having to do with healthcare (such as medical anthropology, medical economics, medical ethics, etc.). The professor will jump at the chance to have students get first-hand experience in a local emergency room. Offer to host a "lab" or "practicum" for students in the course. Each student will take a four-hour shift in your ER once a week. Ideally, you'll have all seven days covered from 4 p.m. to midnight (it's easier than you think to get students to choose the weekend

shifts—they are busier and more exciting). The students get real-life emergency room experience, plus great material for term papers. You get free liaisons (limit the program to juniors and seniors only) who are well-educated, responsible, articulate, and kept in line by their professor who can affect their grades if they don't show up for a shift or who break your behavioral rules (see Press and Smith 1986).

REFERENCES

Becker, H. S., B. Geer, E. C. Hughes, and A. Strauss. 1961. *Boys In White,* 322. Chicago: University of Chicago Press.

Espinosa, J., and L. Kosnik. 1998. "The Overlook Hospital Emergency Department's Journey to Align with the Voices of Its Customers." [Press, Ganey Success Story Entry].

Hall, M., and I. Press. 1996. "Keys To Patient Satisfaction in the Emergency Department: Results of a Multiple Facility Study." *Hospital and Health Services Administration* 41 (4): 515-30.

Mayer, T., and R. Cates. 1998. "Are they Patients or Are they Customers?." *The Satisfaction Monitor* (July/Aug): 1-5.

McCaig, L. F. 1994. "National Hospital Ambulatory Medical Care Survey: 1992 Emergency Department Summary." [Press Release]. Washington, D.C.: NCHS (HHS). March 2.

Press, I., and D. Smith. 1986. "Premedical Students as Patient and Family Liaisons in the Emergency Department: A Strategy for Patient Satisfaction." *Journal of Emergency Nursing* (Jan/Feb): 23-25.

Roth, J. A., and D. J. Douglas. 1983. *No Appt. Necessary.* New York: Irvington Publishers, Inc.

CHAPTER 10

Implementing Change

AN INSTITUTION-WIDE patient satisfaction focus will be more successful than a piecemeal attempt to improve satisfaction. With the broad approach, everyone is brought on board at the same time and pockets of resistance are minimized and readily identifiable. Beginning small or making piecemeal attempts at culture change to "test the waters" indicates a lack of institutional confidence and commitment. This final chapter outlines the steps needed to implement an effective program.

GETTING STARTED

An official, broadly planned, institution-wide plan backed by universal training, discussion, monitoring (measurement), expectations, and rewards is also much easier than a piecemeal attempt. When everyone in the organization reflects and reinforces the values, individuals stay committed. Peer pressure alone will keep things moving. Such group pressures keep cultures going on a day-to-day basis. Resist the temptation to "begin things small and see how it works."

Establish a Context

Begin with a plan. Contact other hospitals to learn what they have done to make patient satisfaction a core element of their culture. Ask, "What has worked and what hasn't? How did they set goals? What rewards and incentives have they used?"

Initiate a major kickoff campaign long before you start holding people accountable for patient satisfaction. First generate internal publicity. Explain what is going to happen, describe the goals, and focus on the advantages for staff, physicians, and patients. Require each group to prepare a written report outlining what they see as their role in the satisfaction culture. You may want to create a campaign name, perhaps an acronym for various attributes you are stressing. For example, Holy Cross Hospital in Chicago named its campaign "SERVE": Service, Excellence, Respect for patients, Value, and Enthusiasm. You can easily invent something similar.

Memorial Hospital Pembroke (Florida) groups its customer service behavioral standards under the headings: professionalism; attitude; teamwork; effective communication; pride; and safety awareness. Each heading became an acronym for the specific standards. Acronyms can be useful as mnemonic devices that help staff remember specific points. For example, "attitude" is broken down into a behavioral standard for each letter of the word.

Attitude makes a difference. Be positive.

Thank each and every customer.

Treat each person as if he or she is the most important person in the organization.

Initiate a connection. Say hello.

Take them there. Escort lost customers.

Understand the customer's needs.

Display appropriate body language.

Exceed our customers' expectations.

Establish a Satisfaction Baseline

Before starting on a patient satisfaction initiative, you should have begun measuring patient satisfaction. If you already have a survey going, your QI teams can practice problem identification and problem solving with the most recent survey results. How will you handle communications with your lowest-scoring nursing unit or department? How can you prevent them from becoming overly defensive? How will you incentivize them to improve? How will goals be established for future improvements?

Control the Metaphor

Management must stress that low satisfaction scores at the beginning of the process are a *challenge* and an *opportunity*—not a problem or occasion for punishment. The idea of linguistically converting "problems" into "opportunities" sounds a lot like spin-doctoring, but it works. What you call something is how you ultimately respond to it. By stressing that low scores are opportunities for improvement and recognition, staff come to view them as challenges and a chance to gather accolades and rewards. In this way, the satisfaction survey becomes a tool rather than a threat.

Leave No One Out!

If you are going to measure their performance, staff have got to be involved from the beginning. Too often we hear of staff who have never seen their survey or data reports, or who did not participate in (or were allowed to bug-out of) initial orientation sessions about patient satisfaction and institutional expectations about performance. This is particularly the case with physicians.

Involve Your Doctors from the First

Ultimately, no satisfaction or quality improvement program can work if the physicians aren't on board. Usually they are the last to buy into the importance of patient satisfaction as a measure of the quality of care. Quite often this lack of buy-in is caused by the physicians not being involved in the culture change program from the beginning. Someone in management says, "The docs won't want this. You know how they are. Let's not involve them until it's working well." With this kind of attitude, the program likely *won't* work well. Physicians' influence (professional, moral, and political) is too pervasive to be ignored. Your survey should contain some items about patient satisfaction with physicians. Make sure physicians are given the opportunity to at least comment on the survey items that involve their interaction with patients. Your chief of staff should be involved in discussions that identify potential causes and courses of action should scores (both in general and for individual physicians) be low. If you have a senior-level patient satisfaction committee, a physician should definitely be on it.

Wabash Valley Practice Management (which manages a number of physician practices in hospitals around Terre Haute, Indiana) at first presented blind patient satisfaction scores to its physicians. No individual was identified, and no progress was made in satisfaction, either. Taking advantage of the competitive nature of physicians, they began identifying individual scores where all physicians could see them. Some "went into denial." For most of the physicians, however, the strategy worked and satisfaction scores improved dramatically. Wabash Management points out that some of the busiest practices (highest patient-to-physician ratio) achieved highest patient satisfaction. This undermines the common excuse that "we have no time to spend on nonessential behaviors."

A note on involving physicians: The chief physician (be it chief of staff, chairman of the medical group, ED director, or whatever) must be on board and must take responsibility for his or her staff's patient satisfaction effort, or it won't work. Only physicians have real credibility with other physicians. The physician leader must speak with low-scoring docs, encouraging a search for possible causes and suggesting possible behavioral or practice changes. The survey manager for the hospital or practice (usually not a physician) should have previously spoken with the leader about possible causes that may be affecting the low-scoring physician's performance. If there are written survey comments, the leader shares these with the physician.

Patient satisfaction must always be an agenda item at medical staff meetings.

Try for Some Early Successes

Do not go for a single, long-term, "all or nothing" goal. Set goals of differing lengths, based on levels of difficulty. Start with a set of easily and quickly achievable score goals. You will generate stronger commitment if you continuously achieve successes along the way. Try to pick some low-hanging fruit. From your patient satisfaction data, select lower-scoring issues whose causes are pretty obvious and not too complex or expensive to address. Fix them. Celebrate the improvement in scores. Publicize it. Give out some rewards.

Prioritize Your Projects

To select targets for quality improvement, go beyond a "priority index," which looks at scores plus the relationship of each item with overall satisfaction. Remember, lower scores and higher correlation with overall satisfaction means higher priorty. Some issues may be of high priority yet are hard or expensive to implement. Target your projects by both priority *and* ease of implementation.

Memorial in Johnstown, Pennsylvania, developed a nine-block grid for prioritizing improvement targets.

First they looked at all of their patient survey questions and judged each issue on whether it would be easy, moderately easy, or

Figure 10.1 Project Prioritization Grid (with Survey Items Allocated to Each)

Relative Ease of Improving

		Easy	Moderately Easy	Difficult
Priority of Issue	**High**	**1** 18, 20, 29, 49	**2** 4, 5, 23, 26, 38, 42	**5** 10, 34, 35
	Medium	**3** 2, 14, 30, 32, 33, 50	**4** 1, 3, 12, 43, 44	**6** 16, 37
	Low	**7** 7, 8, 13, 21, 24, 45, 48	**8** 11, 28, 30, 40, 47	**9** 9, 15, 17, 19, 22, 25, 27, 39, 41, 46

Based on a grid used by Memorial Hospital, Johnstown, Pennsylvania.

difficult to improve. Then they created a priority index of all items on their satisfaction survey and split the list into even thirds which they labeled "high," "medium," and "low" priority. Survey items were then apportioned into the appropriate box. They then did a final prioritization and gave each box a priority ranking (Figure 10.1). The issues in box 1 were to be tackled first (easy-fix "low-hanging fruit" offering quick reinforcement), followed by issues in box 2, then 3, and so forth. The higher the box number, the further in the future improvement was planned. Numbering the boxes is obviously a judgement call, and you might decide to order them differently. This kind of technique helps you to organize your improvement program with more hope of success. Do not pick projects ad hoc. When you rank order them with some logic and structure, it reinforces the validity and utility of your survey data. At the same time, it reinforces the rationale (financial concerns as well as practicality) for your program's targets.

FORMING IMPROVEMENT TEAMS

Ideally, every employee in the hospital—from highest to lowest on the organizational chart—should be on a QI/patient satisfaction team or committee. No matter how modest the function of the team, when someone serves on it, he or she "belongs" and has a stake in furthering the overall mission.

Improvement teams can be formed upon various bases. Memorial Hospital Pembroke in Florida developed the following eight teams for its new program:

1. Inpatient satisfaction
2. Outpatient satisfaction
3. Emergency satisfaction
4. Standards of behavior (for all in the hospital: scripting, etc.)
5. Reward and recognition
6. Service recovery
7. Physician satisfaction
8. Measurement (handling and disseminating the survey and data)

The inpatient satisfaction team, for example, was charged with improving the entire inpatient experience. One area they looked at was admission scores. They developed the following recommendations that were subsequently implemented:

1. Patients are greeted with a smile.
2. All patients are escorted to their area or units.
3. The welcome is scripted.
4. Delays are explained.
5. Waiting areas and lounges are to be renovated.
6. Coffee service is provided.
7. An admitting clerk visits each new patient the day after admission.
8. At this visit, clerk offers any personal care items patient may have forgotten.
9. Staff commit to very best performance at the outset.

Subsequent to their improvement program, overall patient satisfaction with Memorial improved dramatically.

You can create either *situational* teams to tackle ostensibly temporary problems, or *standing* teams to work continually with ongoing issues. If you are undergoing significant construction, a situational "reducing construction irritants team" can work on tactics to reduce inconvenience to patients, and to explain what's going on. If you have low scores for the admitting section of your survey, a situational team can focus on it until the scores rise sufficiently. Many issues are relatively continuous. For example, there will always be complaints and these could be investigated and remedial action recommended by a standing "complaint management team." A "reward and recognition team" could develop and manage hospital-wide rewards for satisfaction score improvement, exemplary service, and so forth.

All hospital-wide teams should consist of members from different departments. Of course, every department and unit should have its own standing patient satisfaction team, charged with monitoring survey results and organizing brainstorming sessions to deal with specific performance issues. All teams should have a percentage of their members rotate off each year, so as to maximize participation (and buy-in) by staff. The existence of specific departmental or unit teams does not preclude the necessity for some hospital-level teams to oversee and support them.

Baptist Health Care in Pensacola created seven hospital-level support teams when they developed their patient satisfaction program. These teams include the:

Measurement Team
Focus: To correctly measure and interpret progress.
  Tasks:
1. Monitor weekly scores and publish results each Thursday. Results are announced in weekly department leader meeting and distributed by e-mail by Thursday afternoon.
2. Identify improvement opportunities.
3. Receive quarterly report from patient satisfaction measurement firm and assist departments in developing improvement plans.

Standards Team
Focus: To create behaviors that support the mission and values.
  Tasks:
1. Develop Standards of Performance manual.
2. Coordinate "Standard of the Month" celebrations throughout hospital.
3. Develop policy that all job applicants must read and sign and agree to honor.

Communication Team
Focus: To develop mechanisms that give all employees access to information about the hospital and its policies.
  Tasks:
1. Develop "communication boards" in each department.
2. Develop agenda for employee forums.

Linkage Team

Focus: To reward and recognize behaviors that align with the standards of performance.

Tasks:

1. Develop hospital-wide and department celebrations for achievements.
2. Develop "champions" program to recognize employees who "go beyond."
3. Develop "legends" program to recognize employees who consistently go beyond.

Irritants Team

Focus: To identify and correct those behaviors, processes, and so forth that irritate our customers.

Tasks:

1. Review available data to determine irritants and develop improvement plans.
2. Initiate and develop service recovery program.

Physician Satisfaction Team

Focus: To build loyalty among physicians and to enhance patient satisfaction with physician services.

Tasks:

1. Create opportunities for dialog with physicians.
2. Include physicians in development of improvement strategies.
3. Measure physician satisfaction with the hospital.
4. Analyze physician suggestions and development improvement plans.

WOW Team

Focus: To develop the tools for staff to reward and recognize each other for living the values.

Task:

1. Develop and monitor the wow card (staff recognizing staff) program.

MONETARY REWARDS FOR DESIRED PERFORMANCE

A number of institutions tie gain-sharing, bonuses, or outright gift-ing to patient satisfaction scores. Typically, satisfaction scores are in the "and if" category ("If profit exceeds one million *and if* patient satisfaction scores place us at least in the 75th percentile vis a vis our peers, then staff will receive ..."). However, the number of hospi-tals and medical practices making patient satisfaction a *leading* cri-terion for monetary rewards is increasing.

Some institutions create a point system, with incremental points awarded for exceeding goals. Thus, in a hospital with a high man-aged care census, the staff bonus pool might be awarded 1 point if average length of stay drops to a particular number, 2 points if that number is even lower, and 3 points if it is below yet another level. Nosocomial infection rate goals might also be divided into three point levels, and so on with other desired and measurable outcomes. Patient satisfaction goals, too, may be divided into three point lev-els. If the minimal target goal for an indicator is not achieved, no points are earned by the staff for that issue. Points are totaled and each is worth a particular dollar amount in bonuses or profit shar-ing. Indicators may be differentially weighted or not.

Monetary awards need not be ongoing (annual, for example). They can be one-shot, to reward staff for having made unprece-dented improvement.

Resist the temptation to "test the waters" by implementing a satisfaction-based monetary award program strictly for senior or middle managers. This can result in significant resentment on the part of nurses and other line staff who do the day-to-day job of treat-ing and serving patients. If you want to start a monetary reward pro-gram piecemeal, begin with the people who actually interact with patients and who are ultimately responsible for their care and sat-isfaction. If they earn their awards, then their managers deserve theirs—but not before.

As indicated earlier, monetary rewards are not essential. You don't need to institute big-buck profit sharing to motivate your staff.

Symbolic rewards work. A personal note from one of the top administrators carries a lot of weight. Whenever top management visits staff and compliments them, whenever a recognition gift is given, whenever top management publicly lauds a department, unit, group, or individual, this constitutes a significant reward.

It cannot be stressed enough that if monetary awards are based at least partially on patient satisfaction, you must provide staff with the training and opportunity to have a positive effect on scores *before* you begin using the data for this purpose. Otherwise, only frustration will result. Setting goals and dangling money in front of them does not help staff actually improve service. Do not confuse *incentives* with *techniques* for improvement! Furthermore, be especially careful to base your reward structure on methodologically sound principles. For example, if you are a medical practice basing physician compensation (or even employment) on satisfaction survey results, you must have a sufficiently large number of returned surveys for each physician to avoid basing action on spurious data.

PUTTING SOME TEETH INTO THE PROGRAM

It's relatively easy to enculturate new employees; they should be hired for patient-focused characteristics they already possess. But what about existing employees, from whom a patient satisfaction program may require new (and possibly threatening) modes of thinking and behaving?

Given the proper introduction, education, preparation, training, and implementation timetable, the vast majority of your existing staff will participate willingly and effectively in your program. However, participation cannot be voluntary—any more than proper hand washing can be left to individual choice. Without teeth, the program won't be taken seriously. If you mean business, those who don't buy in can't stay.

What makes a culture work and sustain itself is that its members *want to* behave as they *have to* behave. But first, you must clearly mandate the "have to's"—the required behaviors. Once your program is running, and once sufficient, realistic "buy-in time" has passed, get rid of those whose unchanged attitudes and behaviors undermine your purpose and commitment. Patients who come into contact with these employees do not deserve less sensitive care than patients who interact with others—the vast majority—of your staff. Tolerating the noncompliant staff members' continued presence visibly suggests that you are not serious.

CONCLUSIONS

It's natural for staff to feel that they are already sensitive to the patient's personal needs and opinions. After all, healthcare naturally selects for such sensitivity, doesn't it? Nonetheless, staff must be "re-educated" in the principles of patient satisfaction and in the specifics of your improvement program. Staff must be primed and involved in the planning, so as to develop ownership in and commitment to the program. The more clearly and specifically your satisfaction program is organized and scripted, the more chance of success.

Also, the more staff actively involved in the program, the more chance of success. Multiple teams or committees (as opposed to a single "satisfaction committee") are advantageous because they broaden the scope of committed employees. If nearly all departments, units, or specialties have their own internal improvement teams, plus at least one member on a hospital-wide team, it makes it more difficult for other department or unit members to opt out of the proper behavioral protocols. Such a strategy puts role models everywhere.

Offering monetary rewards to staff is not really necessary for high patient satisfaction. Rewards are a nice gesture, and if you have the profit to justify it, everyone can use an extra buck, but it is not essential. As we suggested in the very first chapter, patient and employee satisfaction go hand in hand. When staff know they are satisfying patients, they justify and reinforce their own career choice.

Healthcare professionals know that when their customers are satisfied, the result is far more significant than when commodity or other service customers are pleased with the product.

Priority concern for patient satisfaction is not an option for healthcare providers. In an increasingly competitive, litigious, and customer service–oriented economy, satisfying patients is as necessary as infection control and MRI maintenance. When patients are satisfied, what the hospital does to achieve its mission and ensure its survival is reinforced. There is no more cost-effective form of care enhancement, claim prevention, marketing, or employee morale building.

At the same time, given the importance of patient satisfaction as a key component of quality care, as an outcome of care, as a driver of profit, and as an indicator of staff performance, it must be measured correctly. When done right and used right, such measurement becomes an invaluable tool. You win, your patients win, your staff win, your payers win.

Patient satisfaction is good medicine.

And good business.

Index

Halo effect, 67
Hand-outs, 83
Health Plan Employer Data and
    Information Set (HEDIS), 18
Health plans, 11-12
HEDIS. *See* Health Plan Employer Data
    and Information Set
Hopes, 35-36
Hospital causes of dissatisfaction, 140, 142
Humoral medicine beliefs, 43

Identity: acknowledgment, 69-70; threats,
    61-64, 67, 115
Illness: definition, 46-47; evolution,
    47-61; explanatory models,
    51-54; presentation to physician,
    58-61; roles/identities, 61-64; self-
    treatment, 54-56; sick role, 56-58;
    staff interactions, 65; symptoms,
    47-51
Improvement goals, 144-45
Inconvenience threshold, 187-88
Information: believability, 13-14;
    omission, 60
Integrated culture, 155
Interaction, 6, 36-39, 159-61
Interactive voice response (IVR), 83
Interim goals, 146
Internal referents, 146-47
Internet surveys, 82
Interpersonal skills, 21
Irritants team, 228
IVR. *See* Interactive voice response

Labeling patients, 57-58, 69, 194-96
Language barriers, 65
Length of stay, 122-23
Linkage team, 228

Mail-back surveys, 80-81
Malpractice claims, 20-21, 23
Mean scores, 100, 101
Measurement team, 227
Medical management: satisfaction and, 23;
    sick roles and, 69; stress and, 6-7

Medical specialty, 125-26
Medical system as "open" or closed,"
    37-38, 45
Misconceptions, 38-39, 40
Moments of truth, 29-32
Monetary rewards, 229-30, 231
Moral evaluation of patients, 192-94, 207
Multiple variables, 128-31
Multiple-wave mailing, 89, 92

National Committee for Quality
    Assurance (NCQA), 1, 18
National database, utility of, 148
National Quality Forum, 19
NCQA. *See* National Committee for
    Quality Assurance
Negative predisposition and claims, 21
Newsletter, 158, 172-73
Noise, 45
Nonresponse bias, 91-92

Open postcards, 89
Opportunity cost, 11-12
Organization, 140
Organizational rules, 39, 42
Outcome: communication and, 5;
    indicator, 4
Over-survey, 92-93

Pain: variable expression of, 48-49;
    tolerance, 48
Participation rewards, 84
Patient: attitude, 7-8; comments, 143-44,
    148; compliance, 5-6; culture, 38,
    45-46, 67; as customers, 157;
    experience of care, 4; healthcare
    viewpoint, 10-11; identifier, 122, 133;
    labels, 57-58; language use, 60-61;
    liaison, 208, 216; moral legitimacy,
    195; primary needs, 37; tracking
    system, 212; withholding
    information, 60
Patient satisfaction: accountability and,
    18-20; benefits, 1; competitive
    strength, 10-15; definition, 23;

employee satisfaction relationship, 8-10; pledge, 174; profitability and, 15-18; quality of care correlation, 4-8; risk management and, 20-22; value, 24

Patient satisfaction initiative: baseline, 221; context, 220; goals, 223; opportunities, 221; physician involvement, 222-23; priorities, 223-25; staff involvement, 221; tips, 223

Payer, 126-27

Pediatric treatment room, 212

Peer achievement, 145-46

Peer-recognition programs, 166-67

Percentile rank, 148

Perception, 2-3; culture filter, 36-37; patient causes and, 142; of physician competence, 4; placebo effect, 7; reality and, 137-38; satisfaction surveys, 78-80

Performance: expectations, 33-35, 58; internal data and, 119; judgement, 41; rewards, 229-30

Personal issues, 38-39

Personality, 140

Personnel, 140

Physician: accountability, 215; communications, 3, 4; enthusiasm, 7-8; illness presentation, 58-61; interaction, 208; profiling, 127-29; satisfaction team, 228; technical competence, 4

Placebo effect, 7-8

Positive predisposition, 22

Practice management group, 206

Predisposition: experiences and, 29-32; negative, 21; positive, 22; primary care, 186

Priorities, 101, 212-13

Prioritization grid, 224

Priority index: data interpretation, 113-16; for diagnosis-related group, 131-32; grid, 223-24; for quality improvement, 118-19

Privacy issues, 89, 215

Problem patient, 42-43, 57-58

Problem solving, 139-43, 150

Profitability, 15-18

Publicity, 157-58

QI. *See* Quality improvement

Quality improvement (QI): correlation coefficients, 118-19; priority index, 116, 118-19; report cards and, 20, 75-76; targets for, 131-32, 133; teams, 225-28

Quality indicator, 5, 19

Question wording, 136

Quick wins, 211

Real-time surveys, 82-83

Recognition: management, 167-68; peer programs, 166-67; reward mechanisms, 168, 169; samples, 179-81

Recollections, 78-80

Recommendations, 66-67, 198, 200, 203

Reinforcement, 146, 157-58

Report cards: effects, 19; function, 76; quality improvement and, 20, 75-76

Resource utilization, 17-18, 23

Respondents, 187-89, 04

Response bias, 90-91

Response percentages, 101-3

Response rates, 89-90, 92-94

Response scale, 96

Reward and recognition team, 226

Rewards, 214, 229-30, 231-32

Risk management, 20-22

Roles: acknowledgment, 69-70; threats, 61-64, 67, 115

Sampling, 89-90

Satisfaction pool, 214

Satisfaction score, 206, 215

Satisfaction survey: answer scale, 87; appearance, 83-84; cover letter, 84, 85, 96; data limitations, 77; development, 149-50; food questions, 86; grouping questions,

About the Author

A CO-FOUNDER OF Press, Ganey Associates, Irwin Press, Ph.D., was the first to nationally promote patient satisfaction as both a component and indicator of healthcare quality. Since 1985 he has worked with hospitals across the country to implement satisfaction measures and improvement strategies.

Dr. Press received his B.S. in chemistry from Northwestern University, and his Ph.D. in cultural anthropology from the University of Chicago. He has been a professor of anthropology at the University of Notre Dame since joining the faculty in 1965. He has conducted field research in Mexico, Colombia, Spain, and the United States, publishing widely on the clash between alternative ("folk" or "popular") medical practices and clinical ("official") medicine. His investigations into why patients use alternative healers rather than (or in addition to) physicians and formal medicine led to his winning a Lilly Faculty Fellowship and appointment as visiting professor at the University of Miami School of Medicine in 1980. There he spent the year rotating through all clinical services at Jackson Memorial Hospital, observing interactions between patients and staff and recording patients' experience with clinical care.

Since founding Press, Ganey (with Rodney F. Ganey, Ph.D.) in 1985, Dr. Press has devoted himself to the task of making patient satisfaction measurement both practical and useful for physicians, hospitals, and other providers. He has served on the Quality Improvement Taskforce of the Joint Commission on Accreditation of Healthcare Organizations, and is a member of the Research and Quality Improvement Council of the National Quality Forum. A popular keynote speaker and workshop leader, he is widely recognized for his insight into the personal factors that affect the patient's experience and evaluation of care.